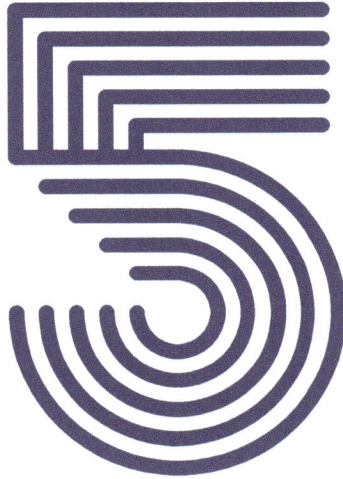

5 FOR LIFE

Healthy ways for healthy weight

MEGAN DYSON

Published by Maireana Press, South Australia

First edition

First published 2022

© Megan Dyson, 2022

ISBN 978-0-6454315-0-6

A catalogue record for this book is available from the National Library of Australia

Cover and interior design by Tess McCabe

Editing by Dr Amy Lovat

Photo by Lucylu Photography

Disclaimer

The information and recommendations contained in this book are intended as general in nature, and are not intended as medical advice or a substitution for medical advice given by a healthcare professional. Readers experiencing any illness or medical condition, including a mental health condition, should consult a medical professional before commencing any weight reduction program or diet.

The author and publisher make no representation, express or implied, as to the accuracy of the information contained in this book, errors or omissions, or the suitability of information or recommendations for any person, and accept no responsibility for any loss or damage suffered by any person acting upon any material contained in this publication.

CONTENTS

PREFACE

When I was growing up, our diet was largely vegetarian. My mum was an excellent cook, so we ate a lot of Mediterranean-style things – stuffed vegetables, moussaka… and a lot of pulses: chickpeas, lentils and dried beans, as well as textured vegetable protein (which we all hated). We had meat now and then, and chicken on special occasions.

After leaving home in my twenties, I became a fan of 'low-fat, high-carb' diets which were popular at the time. I had no idea about different types of carbs, and focused just on fat content, which I was certain was the key to healthy eating.

That was the 1990s, and I wasn't alone. Even when an older and much wiser friend told me firmly that 'eating fat doesn't make you fat', I argued, as an opinionated twenty-something, that he was quite wrong.

What didn't I like about the way my body felt in those days? I carried weight around my hips and thighs, and had a poor digestive system, complete with an intermittent irritable bowel. My energy levels were often very low, and I just felt sluggish a lot of the time.

Becoming pregnant at thirty, I resolved to eat the best for my baby, and started looking more carefully into what I 'should' be eating. The answer was clearly more vegetables, more good fat from nuts and fish, and more protein. So I ate more of these things, and it just didn't leave much room for other food – refined carbs or junk food.

The result was a radical improvement in gut comfort, even with the baby occupying most of the space! After our son was born, I returned to my normal weight – but with leaner hips and thighs, higher energy levels, and real muscle definition, despite not being a big exerciser.

As the pace of life increased with children and starting my own business, I began to slip back into some old ways of eating. It often felt quicker to make a sandwich than a salad for lunch, grab a couple of slices of fruit toast or a muesli bar on the run...

Then about ten years ago, my husband was diagnosed with late onset type 1 diabetes, which brought us face-to-face with the 'carb issue' in a very raw way. It was confronting to realise what a strain we put on our bodies every time we eat carbs; in particular, highly processed, refined carbs like sugar, rice, bread and cake. Our household diet changed once again.

In the years after the diabetes diagnosis, I began to research all things nutrition in earnest.

My day job in environmental law and policy is dense in facts, science and analysis, and I love really getting to the bottom of things. Nothing much I like better than sifting through hunches, suspicions, opinions and research to find evidence, and I complemented my growing knowledge with formal studies in nutrition.

It became clear that what's needed, and what works for improving body composition as well as a healthy attitude towards food, is to build a set of eating habits that play strongly in our favour. There wasn't anything that covered what I see as the five crucial elements of healthy eating, and that was supportive in the way I want to be supported, so I decided to get my ideas down on paper.

I hope the unique approach of *Five for Life* helps you begin to think differently about food and eating, and ultimately to become comfortable and confident in your own body.

INTRODUCTION

This might be the first book you've picked up about healthy eating, or it might be one of many. If you've been looking for a way to reduce weight and body fat, chances are you're already feeling frustrated, overwhelmed or disheartened by conflicting ideas and just too much information.

Bookshops, media and the internet are awash with advice – mostly well-meaning, sometimes cynical, often contradictory, and much of it based on no evidence at all.

'Diet culture' is a vast and lucrative industry, yet it rarely seems to help anyone in the long term.

Part of the reason is that the focus is almost entirely on what to eat, ignoring the fact that we are whole human beings, and that what we eat is only part of the overall picture for healthy eating. To make things worse, the 'what to eat' advice is often unnecessarily prescriptive, confusing or plain incorrect. And there's frequently an unhealthy undercurrent promoting self-judgement and a sense of not being 'enough'.

Five for Life is different. Based on the latest research, it focuses not just on what we eat, but on the why, when, what, how and how much of eating. It's compassionate and grounded in self-acceptance and appreciation for our own unique body.

Using direct and straightforward language, Five for Life is a *simple, evidence-based approach to reducing weight, built around a set of healthy eating habits that anyone can adapt to their own life, for life*. Not just the 'what to eat' bit, but all the threads that together create a healthier approach to food and eating.

In terms of *what* to eat, it's important to know that this isn't a diet book. There are plenty of diet books and diet plans around, often promoting a fad food or single-solution approach.

Ultimately, the best diet is the one you stick with, because it fits your broad food preferences and culture. The Five for Life approach can be applied to any diet that emphasises vegetables (especially greens), limits sugar and other refined carbohydrates, and includes sufficient protein and high-quality fats.

Who's it for?

This book is for people who aren't happy with the weight they're carrying because it's limiting their lifestyles and lives. It's for people who are tired of feeling sluggish or slow, and want to reduce their body fat safely and permanently.

It's not about obsession, self-torture, or perpetuating myths about body shape and self-worth. Beauty has nothing to do with body shape, and it's well past time we broke that artificial nexus.

Our bodies are our very own precious vessels, carrying us through our lives, ideally with dignity, grace and strength. Worthy of our *own* deep love, admiration and support. Other people's opinions are just not relevant.

There are lots of reasons, some complex, some simple, and all highly personal, for why we carry more weight than we'd like. The common thread is **our eating habits: why and when we eat, what we eat (and drink) and how we eat**.

This book is for you if you want to reduce the amount of fat you're carrying, and:

- you're confused by conflicting advice, and no longer sure what you 'should' be eating

- you have a fair idea about healthy diets, but for whatever reason, aren't eating that way

- you are eating the right food, but it seems to make no difference to your weight, or

- you're just interested in learning more about healthy eating.

If you have or suspect you might have an eating disorder, please seek out professional help rather than going it alone with a book about eating habits, even this one.

In some parts of this book, I'm speaking directly to women aged between about 30 and 65. This is because I'm part of that group myself, and very aware of the significant hormonal changes we experience during that period, and how disrupting those changes can be on our lives, including our weight and body shape.

A short word about sex and gender

Some nutrition metrics (e.g. about optimum waist measurements, recommended energy intake and vitamin and mineral needs) are sex-based because of the impact that hormones have on our nutritional requirements and on our metabolism, including the way we burn and store fat. For that reason, this book sometimes includes suggestions of one thing for women, and another for men. If you don't identify in a binary way, or with your sex assigned at birth, choose the suggestion that most closely reflects what your hormones are up to.

Healthy ways for healthy weight

Healthy eating can seem confusing, and it certainly helps perpetuate 'diet culture' to keep us thinking that way! But it turns out that in the end, it's fairly simple.

Unlike diets, which focus only on what to eat, Five for Life is about building habits you can live with, around five pillars of healthy eating – the Five Habits.

1. *Doing it for love – treasuring your body*

2. *Eating at the right time*

3. *Eating the right food*

4. *Drinking the right fluids (water!)*

5. *Eating the right way*

The habits are a set of interdependent behaviours that work together, like pieces of a puzzle. At the centre is the first and most important habit: a mindset that helps remind you why you care – the habit of treasuring your own special body. Cherishing it, and making choices that reflect that.

Slow, steady and sustainable

Weight gain is the result of many weeks, months and years of small choices that eventually become ingrained habits around eating. Weight *reduction* occurs in the same way, so be patient – this is going to take a while.

Changing weight for the better, forever, can only happen by changing the way you think about food and eating. Changes in body composition will follow, but this is definitely not a book about rapid weight reduction, 'miracle weight loss' or 'overnight success'.

Safe and sustainable reduction in body fat will be slow. It will take time for your body to adjust its metabolism to find and maintain new, lower levels of stored fat. Expect to see small differences in weight, shape and mindset over the first month, which will become more noticeable over time.

There (might) be safe ways to shed a lot of weight quickly, but if you haven't adopted new ways of eating to back up weight maintenance once you reach your goal, the strong odds are that you'll regain all the weight you shed, and more, once you return to old habits. Your body will rebel against the imposed 'famine', and strive to carry even higher amounts of fat to keep you safe from future food shortages.

'Other people'

Maybe we all have the friend who seems to eat 'whatever they like' while maintaining a slim build. Or the friend who never eats breakfast, snacks on chocolate biscuits late at night, and likewise never seems to put on weight.

These people are outliers – people who, for genetic reasons, seem to have an extraordinary capacity to hold their body at a low and lean set point, regardless of what they eat. They might always be like this; it's also possible that one day their genetic switch will be flicked, and things will change. Meanwhile, if their eating habits haven't been successful for you, don't be disheartened – you're just like the rest of us!

Eating vs. exercise

The most important contributor to our weight (specifically, body fat) is what we put in our mouth, not how much we exercise – in fact, what we eat and drink is about 80% of what matters. On average, 10–20% of our 'energy out' goes to physical activity, including everyday movement as well as deliberate exercise. We use the rest of our energy just maintaining bodily systems, including digestion, and we have relatively little control over that.

But we do control 100% of the 'energy in' – *what we put in our mouth, and when.*

Adequate exercise is essential for good health, but without changing our eating habits, exercise will not bring us to a healthy weight, and it can't compensate for poor eating habits.

That's why this book is about eating, not exercise. *The single most significant thing we can do to reach and keep a healthy weight is to change our eating habits.*

Weight vs. body composition

Throughout this book, when I mention 'weight', it's shorthand for *body composition*. Our weight is made up of fat, muscle, bone, water, blood and organs. When we say we want to reduce weight, what we really mean is that we want to *reduce the part of our weight that is body fat*. But that's a real mouthful, so I'll just talk about reducing weight. Now and then I'll add a reminder that we're talking about reducing the fat part of that weight.

Finding your way around the book

The book is designed to be read from front to back, but you can dip into it at any point.

Part I introduces the Five Habits, with suggestions for how to cement them into your daily life. Each of these chapters include some ideas for reflection, too – a series of questions to help you identify where and how you might make direct changes in your own life. I suggest keeping a journal or other written habit helper, to jot down your thoughts.

Part II looks at some important topics that cut across the Five Habits – the three M's (micronutrients, microbiome, metabolism) and the three S's (stress, sleep, shift work). It also has a chapter on the special challenges that women face during and after pregnancy and menopause.

Part III is about using the habits to help make changes in day-to-day life – whether that's living with younger children, getting home late after a long day at work, eating out or socialising with friends.

By the end of the book, you'll have collected a toolbox of new ways to think and act, which will help bring you towards your own weight goal.

If you're interested in more detail or further reading, the References section at the back lists some of the research resources.

All you need

✓ An open mind and willingness to learn.

✓ Bathroom scales (digital) and a measuring tape (cloth or plastic).

✓ A journal, notebook and pen, or an electronic device for writing.

What you don't need...

You don't need anything else! I won't be asking you to:

✗ count calories

✗ eat special things, or buy pills or supplements

✗ cut out food groups, or combine foods in any particular way

✗ use any special equipment

✗ spend money on ongoing support or coaching

✗ commit lots of time.

And you don't need 'willpower', either. You're just going to learn new habits, and unlearn some old ones.

If you want an overview before you start, or a quick reminder of key points at any time, have a look at *Five for Life – the short story* below, or download it from the Five for Life website (a QR code link to the website is on the back cover).

Five for Life – the short story

To reach and keep a healthy weight, we need to reduce body fat safely and keep it off permanently, without losing muscle mass or bone density, and without feeling hungry or deprived.

To achieve this, we need first to understand our own reasons for wanting to change our body shape and what stands in our way, then make a commitment to a new approach. Gradually building up our own set of supportive habits, the Five for Life approach to food and eating becomes an easy part of our everyday routines.

The Five Habits, explained in detail in Part I, are:

1. The right motivation – treasure your body

- Look after your precious body – it's the only one you have.

- Understand why you want to change your weight, and identify your barriers.

- Set a goal and keep your eye on it. Regularly track progress. Commit to practising some healthy eating habits every day.
- Mind your language and behaviour – you're not 'on a diet'.
- Stay physically active – for joy and general health. But know that weight reduction and maintenance is mostly about changing the way you eat.
- Manage stress and get enough sleep.

2. *The right time*

- Identify the reasons why, apart from hunger, you eat. Recognise and challenge them.
- Eat in sync with your circadian rhythm (internal body clock). This means eat early: have breakfast every day, and finish eating at least three to four hours before going to bed.
- Be aware of portion sizes, and eat a small meal regularly.
- Consume most of your energy before 3 pm and significantly reduce the size of your last meal of the day.

3. *The right food*

- Eat a lot more vegetables, especially greens and other non-starchy vegetables.
- Eat more protein, including vegetarian protein, and good-quality fats from natural sources such as nuts and seeds, fish and cold-pressed oils.
- Eat less high-carb, high-starch food, including potatoes, rice, bread, pasta and noodles. Eat less refined vegetable oil and processed fat: it's in most processed food and deep-fried food.
- Avoid or eat rarely and with care:
  » sugar, including sweetened drinks, fruit juice, lollies and sweets
  » highly processed food such as food made with refined flour and processed cereals, most processed meats and packaged meals, and artificial sweeteners

» 'danger zone' foods – starchy carbs prepared with fat and sugar (e.g. cake, chocolate, pastries and desserts) or with fat and salt (e.g. pizza, chips and crisps).

4. The right fluids

- Drink more water – aim for at least three litres of plain water every day. Herbal tea counts too.

- Drink less caffeine and alcohol.

- Avoid soft drinks (whether sweetened with sugar or artificially), vitamin waters, energy drinks, sports drinks, flavoured milk and fruit juice (even if it has no added sugar).

5. The right way

- Savour food. Consider its origins and acknowledge its significance in your life.

- Pay attention. Mindful eating helps us enjoy food more and prevents overeating.

- Chew slowly and thoroughly, making the meal last.

- Keep a food journal for a few days every month or so, to better understand what you eat, when, why and how.

PART I

THE FIVE HABITS

This part starts with a chapter about habits and how to change them, then sets out the pillars of healthy eating: the Five Habits.

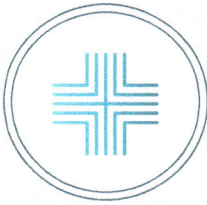

CHAPTER ONE.
CHANGING HABITS

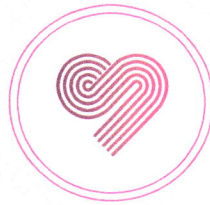

CHAPTER TWO.
TREASURE YOUR BODY

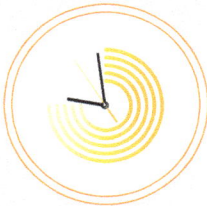

CHAPTER THREE.
WHEN TO EAT

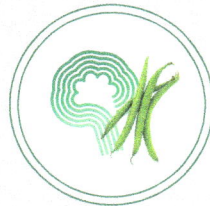

CHAPTER FOUR.
WHAT TO EAT

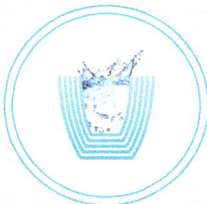

CHAPTER FIVE.
WHAT TO DRINK

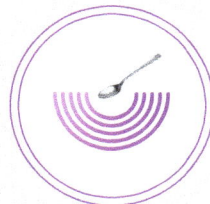

CHAPTER SIX.
HOW TO EAT

CHAPTER ONE

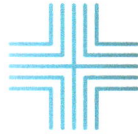

CHANGING HABITS

The way we think about food and eating, whether consciously or not, plays out in the way we eat: that is, our *eating habits*. So, the only way to make permanent change in our weight is to change those habits.

What will it take?

The first step in changing an unhelpful habit is to notice it… notice that it's weighing us down, and gain insight into what triggers it. Because most habits are unconscious, this first step is the most important, and can also be the most difficult. Why have we formed this habit? What sets the behaviour in motion? What 'rewards' are wrapped up in this habit (especially the common habit of eating when we aren't hungry)?

The second step is to work out how to disrupt the sequence with new behaviours. Substituting a different routine, or a different reward, is one way to do this. For example, if the habit is having a sweet something with your morning coffee, you could change to a pot of tea and a chat with a friend, or decide coffee goes better with a piece of fruit.

The last step is dismantling the old habit loop by practising the new habits.

Establishing new habits takes a conscious commitment to continual practice. It also takes time.

Your current eating habits have probably been with you for many years, some even since childhood, so be patient and persistent to help the changes stick. Research suggests that new eating patterns can be formed within three weeks, but it takes daily conscious repetition over 10 weeks or so to embed them into our everyday routine. Each time we repeat an action, *we are more likely to perform that same action again in the future.* Each repetition of a new behaviour brings it closer to being a natural reflex.

In this book, I introduce the five core behaviours at the heart of Five for Life, as well as lots of small actions and strategies for making them stick. I call these the *habit helpers*, and they're set inside the shaded boxes. You don't need to do all these things at once and all of the time! Think of them as tools to help you change, and add a few new ones each week. There's no rush. The only way to shed excess weight safely and permanently is to change the way you think and feel about food and eating, by steadily building a set of behaviours that will last.

Incremental tool kit

Start small. Choose two or three things to change and make them a solid part of your daily routines before adding a few more. By incrementally building up strong habits, they eventually become second nature without us getting overwhelmed.

You could write down your choices each week and stick them to the fridge or next to your desk. Use sticky notes in the side of this book to mark ideas that really resonate with you, or jot things down in a notebook or on your computer. Or make a list of things you'll do with a daily 'tick-sheet' for the week, and mark them off as you go.

Piggyback

Connecting new habits to other activities is a good way to make new habits stick: this is the 'context' or 'habit-stacking' approach. The idea is to join a new habit to something we already do at a certain time (e.g. as part of our morning routine), or in a particular place (e.g. in the car when we put on our seatbelt, or when we sit down at our desk).

Chapters 10 and 11 look at different ways to use the context approach and other tools to develop healthier habits, and shed unhelpful ones.

What are we up against?

It's important to understand what we're up against in terms of developing healthy eating habits; recognising these factors gives us the power to push back against them. Not only are there personal barriers, but our environment itself plays a significant role. The next chapter has more detail about environmental pressures and genetic influences, with tips on how to recognise and protect against these factors throughout the book.

Changing our body composition means changing *why, when, what and how we eat and drink*. In terms of the 'what', there's a blunt truth:

> *If you continue to eat food that is high in processed starch or sugars, your weight will continue to rise.*[1]

To relieve yourself of excess body fat, you must drastically reduce processed starch and sugar: the obvious things like sweets, cake, dessert, pastries, chips and pizza, but also white rice and fruit juice, and bread, pasta and cereal made from refined flours. Although this is only part of the 'what to eat' picture, *it's probably the most important*. Chapter 4 is all about the 'what' of eating.

---

[1] If you're thinking 'but what if I just exercise more?' skip to the section *What about 'calories in − calories out'?* in the next chapter.

Making choices

We are active participants in our own health, never casual observers or bystanders. The choices we make about what we put in our mouths have consequences. This doesn't mean eating a 'perfect' diet all the time; nobody does, and nor should we want that. It just means becoming more aware, and practising conscious choices. And if those choices are sometimes unhealthful, it means accepting that they aren't a mark of moral worth. So no catastrophising or blaming.

What are you waiting for?

Each time we eat or drink, we have the chance to practise a healthy eating habit. What are you waiting for? If not today, when? Are you waiting for this busy patch of work to be over? Waiting until things have settled down at home? Until exams are finished? Until you're well again? Until the baby is born?

There's no point waiting. Healthy eating habits can be started at any time. You don't need to practise everything perfectly every day – just **start small, stay steady, and build up**. Do at least one thing, every day.

Journaling

While you're going through this book, building up your own store of new habits, a journal is an excellent tool.

Working out why you're not the weight you want to be, and how you'll change that, means looking quite profoundly inside yourself. You don't need to write that stuff down, but journaling is a good way to gain insight and make the things we learn really stick. It's a powerful tool for understanding our own eating habits and the changes we need to make, and for helping us remember and reinforce our commitments.

The next five chapters include a series of questions ('Reflections', set in boxes) to help you explore how you might put changes into practice. Thinking deeply about the questions will help identify the most important areas for change; of course, these will be different for everyone.

At this stage, you're probably thinking either *Yep, happy to keep a journal*, or *There's no way I'm keeping a journal!* If you're in the second category, you still need something, such as a notebook or computer, so you can get the most out of this book: to record your weight and measurements, and how they change over time as you learn and practise new habits. You'll also need somewhere to jot down things like how much protein you need each day and what you'll do to meet those requirements. Somewhere to keep a food diary too, for at least one week. And quite a few other bits and pieces. It's helpful, trust me.

CHAPTER TWO

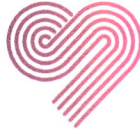

TREASURE YOUR BODY

In this chapter, we go straight to the main point, and the first of the Five Habits. *It's all about you.* What you want, and why. Your body deserves your utmost love and respect. It's the only one you'll ever have, and it deserves to be cherished and nurtured.

This chapter is all about loving your body – your precious vessel.

- *Know why* you want to change, understand your barriers and be kind.
- *Know where* you want to be heading, set your goal and measure progress.
- *Move more*, and stand up straight.
- *Manage stress and get enough sleep*.

Loving your body – the only one you have

An act of love

Our bodies perform an incredible service, every day. Our hips and knees, feet and ankles, carry tens of kilos, lugging them about on uneven surfaces, into and out of different positions. They carry our bags and shopping, and our children too. The more we weigh, the harder they work.

Our heart pumps about five litres of blood every minute throughout our whole body. The bigger we are, the harder our heart must work.

And if we're mothers, then on top of all this, our body has conceived, carried, borne and nurtured our children – it's awe-inspiring!

This faithful body needs and deserves our love, admiration and support. ***It's the only one we'll ever have.*** Be loyal to it.

Becoming and keeping a healthy weight is an act of love. Everything we put in our mouth has a direct impact on our body and its ability to keep serving us – we're the only ones who control what we put in our mouths.

Choose to *live* your love for yourself.

Commit to practice every day

Changing habits means making a commitment to doing something different and fulfilling that commitment each day. It doesn't mean you need to 'do' all the habits straight away and all the time. Just make a promise to yourself to practise the Five for Life approach *in some way, every day*.

- Write down your commitment, and stick it somewhere you'll see it first thing, as well as at other times during the day. Beside your bathroom mirror? On the fridge, in your wallet, on your phone screen? It might be a simple and general prompt (like 'Remember the Five'), or something more specific to the particular habit you want to focus on, such as 'Finish eating by 4 pm today'.

- Each day, look in the mirror and repeat the promise to yourself.
- Let curiosity be your friend. Each day, check in with how you went – what's working, what isn't, how are you feeling about it? Write it down.

Promising someone that you will do something is another way to create an accountability loop that commits you to follow up and helps keep you on track. Choose someone you care about, and whose support you trust. Explain what you're doing and why. Promise regular fortnightly updates and keep faith with it.

Be patient, not perfect

Changing eating habits is a ***slow and cumulative process***. New habits will accrue over time, building a stronger framework as the months go by.

Some days or weeks will be more successful than others. Accept this, and remember that every day is a new opportunity to do something differently. Be patient and kind to yourself.

Feel the love

Showing care and affection for yourself can be difficult, and feel strange. You may have been taught that it's selfish. Time to learn something new.

Every day, we touch our own body hundreds of times – as we get dressed, when we wash our face, clean our teeth and brush our hair. We usually don't give it a second thought. Or maybe we're rough because we're in a hurry. Next time, touch gently, kindly. Acknowledge your *self*.

Language matters – speak kindly

We can be our own worst enemies when it comes to treasuring our bodies, in the things we say about or to ourselves, or allow others to say to us.

Listen carefully to the words you use to talk to yourself, or that other people use. What judgements or assumptions do those words carry? Do you ever think or talk about your body as if it's been bad? As if you don't like it? As if it isn't deserving of your utmost respect and care?

You love yourself – so speak kindly to the one you love. In the language you use when you talk about yourself to other people, and the things you say to yourself in your head.

Hang out with people who speak kindly to you, about you, about themselves and about others. You'll feel happier.

Power of words

To create new habits in the language you use to and about yourself, think about what words mean and the feelings they carry. Be truthful in how you use words that are loaded with special meanings.

What positive changes can you make in the language you use and the way you speak to yourself?

For example…

Becoming a healthy eater doesn't mean you'll 'lose' weight. Loss is a word that's often heavy with a sense of sorrow or regret. Cherishing your body, feeding it the things it needs and keeping it safe from harm is an act of love. It's joyful.

Healthy eaters aren't on a 'diet'. Dieting carries negative connotations for many of us. A 'diet' can be the thing that never works; that's expensive or time-consuming; or that involves special food, weighing things and feeling hungry. A diet can seem to take you further away from how you want to live your life, not closer. The Five for Life way is not a diet. Eating healthily is a gift you give this precious vessel you call your body. This body that will carry and sustain you for the rest of your life.

Liberation – not deprivation

Healthy eating habits are in no way a form of deprivation. They are true liberation – liberating you from the effects of food advertising, from sugar cravings, from fluctuations in blood sugar, from dysfunctional gut flora – and from the metabolic disorders and excess body fat that go with those things.

Tricks of the mind – language of empowerment

Grappling with kicking the sugar habit, or the chips, or the beer? Studies show that using empowered language, both as self-talk and when we speak to others, changes our mindset in a way that's remarkably motivating. Think – *'I choose to be free of that'* (not *'I am forbidden that'*) or *'I don't eat that'* (not *'I can't eat that'*). *'Not just now thanks, maybe later'* (not *'I'm on a diet'*).

HABIT HELPERS – LOVE

Picture it. Visualise your body as a perfectly designed and built, finely tuned machine (it is). It needs the very best-quality fuel, in the right amounts, and at the right time.

The only one, ever. Treat your body as though it's the only one you'll *ever* have (it is). As you go about your day-to-day activities, tend your body gently, with care.

Choose love. Looking after your precious body is an act of love. Each time you eat or drink is an opportunity to make that real.

Commitment. Commit to make small changes, every day. Slow and steady. No need to get everything right (not today, and not ever), but no reason to wait either. Build change slowly and steadily. Aim for practice, not perfection.

Kindness. Make a note of kind and appreciative words that describe you. Use them.

Think it; say it. Shedding excess fat is a joyful process of liberation, not loss. Change your perspective and the words you use (in your head and aloud) – *__don't, not can't__. Liberation, not deprivation!*

What are you looking for, and why?

Carrying excess fat isn't healthy. It's strongly linked to a range of diseases including type 2 diabetes, metabolic syndrome, non-alcoholic fatty liver, heart disease, and 13 different types of cancer. But 'knowing' this stuff isn't the same as it being meaningful enough to make lasting changes to our lifestyle.

The weight we are, and the weight we want to be, are intensely personal subjects. We're unlikely to reach and keep our ideal weight and body composition unless we understand and deeply acknowledge why we're not the way we want to be.

Think about these questions – you also might like to make notes in your journal.

If the *only* reasons you aren't happy with your weight stem from the opinions of other people, including the media, it's important to acknowledge that, and to make a stand for yourself against external pressures. Healthy eating habits will benefit you for the rest of your life, regardless of your preferred body shape, so do keep reading this book! But if you don't want to reduce weight, some parts, including sections in this chapter on choosing targets and monitoring progress, won't be applicable.

Loving yourself

You are a whole and multi-faceted human being. You're not defined by your body – its shape or size. You aren't your appearance. You're not somehow a 'version' of yourself. Separate your love and respect for yourself from how you perceive your body shape, or what you weigh.

Consider what you admire and appreciate about yourself, just as you are right now. Maybe it's your positive outlook, friendly smile or sense of humour. Your supple skin, bright eyes or glossy hair. Your ability to stand in someone else's shoes. Or your strength and persistence. Why are these things important to you?

Ask yourself whether reducing weight would take any of this away. If you think it might, look more closely at why. What might happen if those things were no longer part of your life?

Not loving your weight

Presumably, you picked up this book because you aren't satisfied with your weight. It's important to identify why you don't like your weight, and exactly what is it that you want to change.

We're confronted, constantly and from an early age, with messages about the 'acceptable' way to look and behave. It's quite likely that part of how you feel about your weight or shape is due to these influences, and it can be difficult to get a balanced appreciation of what really matters.

If you don't like the weight you carry, why? Does it cause you physical difficulties, emotional difficulties, or both? Think about whether any of the reasons 'why' are because of things other people have told you, or that you've read or seen, and whether there's any reason to believe those things. Reasons for changing your weight need to be your own, not someone else's.

Your happy weight

We all have an idea of our 'right weight'. Maybe it's the weight we were before children, or when we played netball or soccer three times a week, or when we last wore our favourite jeans, or at a happier time in our life.

Our best weight is a weight our body is at peace with; it's both objective (what are the health risks?) and subjective (how do I feel?). We each need to make our own choice.

Later in this chapter we look at the objective part of the question, but for now, think about what you identify as your ideal weight, and why. What image of yourself is connected to that sense of an ideal weight? What do you feel would be different or better about your life at that weight?

Understanding barriers

There are probably many reasons why you aren't at your happy weight. Some will be simple; others might be more complex, mental or emotional reasons.

- Maybe your own parents and family didn't have healthy eating habits, so you grew up without the information you needed.

- Maybe you think you need strong willpower to change your eating habits.

- Maybe deep down, changing the shape of your body brings up other fears about change.

- Maybe you think people might belittle you for wanting to make changes, or try to stop you from changing, or love you less.

- Maybe you feel you don't have enough time to prepare healthy meals, or that it will be more expensive than the way you eat now. Or maybe you're concerned that the person who does most of the cooking in your home won't support your changes.

Why are you not your ideal weight? What stops you from being that weight? If you're using a journal, write it down. Be as specific as you can.

Our obesogenic environment

On top of your personal circumstances, there's another likely culprit for why you're not the weight you want to be. According to the Australian Institute of Health and Welfare, our environment is officially 'obesogenic': our surroundings are contributing to overweight and obesity.[2]

We are surrounded by subtle and not-so-subtle messages that it's fine to eat what we like, when we like, and as much as we like. And that the food we are most likely to *like* will be purchased from a shop, not made at home. These messages are brought to you by what we might call 'Big Food'.

---

[2]   Australian Institute of Health and Welfare (2020) Overweight and obesity: an interactive insight.

We're also spending longer hours at work, and less time being physically active when we're not at work, than in generations past.

Our 24-hour-a-day society means that many of us work shifts to feed the beast – in factories and 24-hour service stations, on road works and transport, as journalists, in hospitals and as first-responders. Shift work wreaks havoc with our metabolism, dramatically increasing the likelihood of adding more fat to our frame.

There are other environmental factors at play too, including wider availability of poor-quality food at the expense of good-quality food, and loss of cooking skills. Toxins in the environment, such as endocrine-disrupting chemicals, are also likely to play a part in overweight and obesity.

Chapter 8 explores the effects of stress and lack of sleep, both by-products of modern lifestyles. Chapter 12 takes a look at the role of food advertising, which is an ever-present obesogenic pressure.

What about genes?

It's true that genes play a role in our weight.

Many people carry gene combinations that increase the likelihood of overeating or being highly attracted to the type of food most likely to cause weight gain, and to storing excess fat in dangerous places (within and around our liver, heart and other organs). Additionally, factors in our own lives or our parents' lives even before we were born can switch certain genes on or off. This switching ('epigenetics') can affect our risk of weight gain. Being overweight or obese is also associated with epigenetic changes that increase the risk of developing type 2 diabetes and other diseases.

But being predisposed to something doesn't seal our fate. It's not our destiny. For example, we might have a strong family history of breast or bowel cancer. This doesn't mean that we will get cancer, and there are things we can do to minimise our chances of developing it – like not smoking, reducing alcohol intake, and maintaining a healthy body weight. The same goes for genetic and epigenetic risks of gaining weight.

Self-protection

How do we protect ourselves from obesogenicity and genetic predisposition? It takes *awareness*, *planning* and *determination*.

For genetic risks, think about your own and your family's history or talk to your doctor to find out more. As for the obesogenic environment – it's all around us and that's not likely to change. We need to learn to recognise and notice obesogenic factors in our surroundings, and live safely with them.

Five for Life helps identify steps you can take to protect yourself against risks of weight gain.

HABIT HELPERS – WHAT ARE YOU LOOKING FOR?

Keep your eye on the why. Your motivation to change must come from within. Identify your own reasons, write them down, and remind yourself of them often.

Face up to it. Get a clear view of your own barriers to change, and commit to breaking them down.

'Ideal' weight – where are you heading?

When we decide to change something important about our life, it helps to know exactly where we want to be heading. This section and the next are about how to choose targets that are right for you, and how to measure progress.

Any targets must be motivated by compassion and self-care, as just discussed. They must also be based on good information. This section looks at the difference between body weight and body composition, and how to use both types of information to develop your own targets.

Estimating targets for weight and body fat

In this book, 'reducing weight' is shorthand for *reducing that part of our weight that is body fat.*

So, how can you figure out how much of your weight is body fat? Unless you have regular access to body composition measuring devices (some gyms offer this service), you won't know for sure.

To estimate a target range for healthy weight and body fat with just ordinary bathroom scales and a tape measure, we'll use *a combination of body mass index (BMI) and middle (waist) measurement*. Both of these are only rough estimates, but they're a good and reliable place to start.

BMI doesn't tell us how much of our weight is bone, how much is muscle, how much is water, and how much is fat. But it does give a ball-park idea of whether we're likely to be too heavy for our frame.

Middle (waist) measurement is a much better indicator of body fat, and it's body fat, especially fat held around our middle, that matters the most in terms of health risks.

BMI

The BMI is the ratio of our weight to height. A BMI above the recommended range is associated with increased risk of heart disease, type 2 diabetes, high blood pressure, sleep apnoea and some cancers, as well as increased stress on joints. The higher our BMI is above the recommended range, the greater the health risks.

Step 1: Height

Get a tape measure and measure your height. Even if you think you know how tall you are – let's get accurate.

Get someone to help by placing a book upright on your head. The short edge of the book is resting lightly on the top of your head, the long edge is at right angles against the wall, or a door frame. Mark where the bottom of the book meets the wall with a pencil. Now measure the height from the floor to the pencil mark.

Step 2: Weight

Weigh yourself in the morning when you get up – naked, after you've urinated and before you drink anything. This will be your baseline. This is the weight you measure progress against as you move towards your ideal weight. Always weigh using the same method, at the same time of day.

Step 3: Calculate

Calculate your BMI by putting the numbers into the equation: *weight in kilograms ÷ height in metres squared*. For example, if you weigh 68 kg and you're 165 cm tall, calculate: *68 ÷ [1.65 x 1.65] = BMI 25*.

Alternatively, just enter your height and weight into any online BMI calculator; they all use the correct formula.

Step 4: Record

Write your weight and BMI into your journal or wherever you've decided to record it, with today's date.

Middle measurement

A good indicator of healthy body composition is our middle circumference, across the belly button (navel). This is because the fat that collects on our trunk, around and inside our internal organs, including our heart and liver (known as *visceral fat*), is the most dangerous type of fat and the hardest to lose.

Visceral fat

Visceral fat is sometimes referred to as 'toxic' fat because it produces hormones and other chemicals that travel through the bloodstream, increasing our risk of serious illness including heart disease, type 2 diabetes and some cancers. In women, it is highly associated with breast cancer post menopause, and has also been linked to poor bone health.

As a rough rule, aim for a waist circumference that is less than half your height. More than this increases your risk of developing serious illness.

As hormones dictate where we store fat, including visceral fat, the specific recommendations for middle measurements are:

- Women – *less than 80 cm.*

- Men – *less than 94 cm* (or 90 cm for South Asian, Chinese, Japanese or African Caribbean ethnicity).

If you don't identify with your birth-assigned sex, aim for a waist measurement that's most appropriate for your hormonal status.

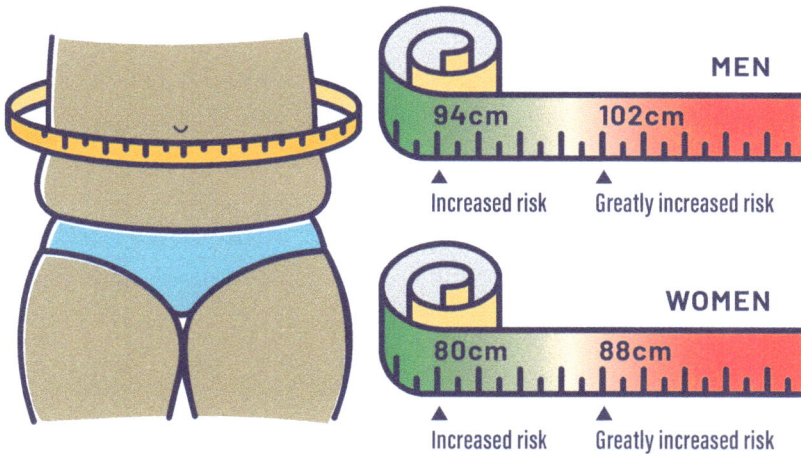

MEN

94cm   102cm

▲ Increased risk   ▲ Greatly increased risk

WOMEN

80cm   88cm

▲ Increased risk   ▲ Greatly increased risk

Step 1: Let's do it

Find your middle – halfway between the top of your pelvic bone and the bottom of your ribs, roughly across your belly button. It won't necessarily be the narrowest part of your torso.

Stand straight, and breathe out. Take the measurement with the tape firmly against your skin, but not digging in.

Step 2: Record

Write down your middle measurement with today's date, alongside your BMI.

How do you know what is *your* best weight?

Every body is a different shape and build. Fat and muscle are differently distributed. Muscle is more compact than fat, so it takes up less space on our body. This means a person carrying a high amount of body fat will look bigger than someone who weighs exactly the same but is carrying more muscle and less fat.

Youth plays a part too – young people tend to have denser, heavier bones than older people, especially women over 50.

You're at your ideal weight when you're in healthy equilibrium. You will be somewhere within the 'low-risk' BMI range **and** your waist measurement will be less than the recommended maximum. And you'll feel good about it.

The BMI gives plenty of scope for ideal weights. A low-risk BMI is considered to be between 18.5 and 25. In terms of kilograms, it's a wide range – a leeway of up to 20 kg, depending on your height. For example, if you're the height of an average Australian woman (165 cm), the BMI 'healthy' range is 51–68 kg, or 17 kilos of choice. Plenty of room for people of all shapes, sizes, ethnicities and ages.

At your ideal weight…

- You'll feel free, joyful and full of energy. You'll have a sense of treading lightly on the earth.
- You won't feel sluggish or lethargic. You won't feel sleepy or heavy after meals.
- You'll find it easy to keep your waist measurement in the healthy zone and your weight within a couple of kilos of your ideal, just by following the healthy eating habits.

Choosing a target weight

If you're above the recommended BMI range

For now, start with bringing your weight within the lower risk weight range (BMI 25 or less).

If you're more than 10 kg above the recommended range, a BMI of 25 is your longer-term goal. You also need some shorter-term goals. Set a mini target of one BMI unit below where you are now. That's around 2–4 kg lighter, depending on your height. Once you're there, aim for the next lower BMI unit.

If you're within the recommended BMI range

If you're already within the lower risk range but it's not your ideal weight, aim for one BMI unit below where you are now (but still within the recommended healthy range), and see how that feels.

If you're below the recommended BMI range

Carrying too little weight (or too little body fat) can also put you at risk of a range of health problems, including reduced bone density, fatigue and lower immune function. If you're below the recommended BMI range, talk to your doctor about the reasons why, and whether this presents mental or physical health risks for you. Only continue with this book on medical advice.

Use the BMI chart on the next page to help find a target weight that's right for you.

Height isn't on the chart? If you're taller than 193 cm, or smaller than 147 cm, you might be feeling left out. The physiological assumptions behind the BMI don't work for heights outside of this range, underestimating BMI for taller people, and overestimating it for smaller people. Talk to your doctor or a dietitian about an appropriate weight range, and use the tape measure method to estimate safe body fat.

Target waist measurements

You'll probably find that one kilogram on the scales correlates to about 1 cm around your waist. Your first target is to reach the maximum recommended waist measurement, then to move below it. If you're more than 10 cm over, set a mini target of 2–4 cm less than your current measurement.

BMI value	LOWER RISK (RECOMMENDED)						INCREASED RISK (OVERWEIGHT)					MODERATE TO SEVERE RISK (OBESE)					
HEIGHT (cm)	19	20	21	22	23	24	25	26	27	28	29	30	31	32	33	34	35
										WEIGHT (kg)							
147	41	44	45	48	50	52	54	56	59	61	63	65	67	69	72	73	76
150	43	45	47	49	52	54	56	58	60	63	65	67	69	72	74	76	78
152	44	46	49	51	54	56	58	60	63	65	67	69	72	74	76	79	81
155	45	48	50	53	55	57	60	62	65	67	69	72	74	77	79	82	84
157	47	49	52	54	57	59	62	64	67	69	72	74	77	79	82	84	87
160	49	51	54	56	59	61	64	66	69	72	74	77	79	82	84	87	89
163	50	53	55	58	61	64	66	68	71	74	77	79	82	84	87	89	93
165	52	54	57	60	63	65	68	71	73	76	79	82	84	87	90	93	95
168	54	56	59	62	64	67	70	73	76	78	81	84	87	90	93	95	98
170	55	57	61	64	66	69	72	75	78	81	84	87	90	93	96	98	101
172	57	59	63	65	68	72	74	78	80	83	86	89	92	95	98	101	104
175	58	61	64	68	70	73	77	80	83	86	89	92	95	98	101	104	107
178	60	63	66	69	73	76	79	82	85	88	92	95	98	101	104	107	110
180	62	65	68	71	75	78	81	84	88	91	94	98	101	104	107	110	113
183	64	67	70	73	77	80	83	87	90	93	97	100	103	107	110	113	117
185	65	68	72	75	79	83	86	89	93	96	99	103	107	110	113	117	120
188	67	70	74	78	81	84	88	92	95	99	102	106	109	113	116	120	123
191	69	73	76	80	83	87	91	94	98	102	105	109	112	116	120	123	127
193	71	74	78	82	86	89	93	97	100	104	108	112	115	119	123	127	130

Write it down

Record your target weight, waist measurement and mini targets, if you're using them, in your journal or notebook.

You might have other goals in mind – like fitting a particular dress or pair of jeans, or being able to reach your shoelaces comfortably. Make a note of these too.

HABIT HELPERS – CHOOSING TARGETS

Avoid comparisons. You don't want to 'look like' someone else, and it's not possible anyway. Our own body, at a particular weight, BMI and fat proportion, will be a different shape from someone else's body at the same weight, BMI and fat proportion. *You will always look like you, and that is a beautiful thing.*

Be realistic. Expect to reduce weight by around 2 kg per month *at most*. We're talking about safe and long-term change, not an overnight metamorphosis.

Be kind. Set mini targets if your ultimate goal feels too daunting.

Measuring progress

Measure with the right mindset

Probably the most important thing to mention about this section before we get stuck in, is that *measuring is a tool for you.*

Setting targets, keeping measurements and actively paying attention to changes help us to monitor progress and identify when we need to make adjustments, and can also help motivate us. But they are only that.

So the rule for this section is: *Weigh and measure with a curious, loving mind.* You're doing this to understand more about how your body responds to changes in eating habits. *You are not weighing in judgement of yourself.*

If you recognise in yourself a tendency to obsessive or perfectionist behaviour, or self-evaluation that produces unhelpful thinking, or if you have or suspect you might have an eating disorder, or if for any reason you don't feel confident to collect and use data in a way that serves your best health – *this section might not be for you*. Weighing and measuring is only safe and worth doing if you find it interesting or motivating, and if you're using the information in a non-judgemental way.

Body weight and shape

To notice and understand the changes in body shape that occur while you're making small changes in habits and lifestyle, it helps to have a reliable baseline. This means you can regularly check in to see what's changing over the weeks and months.

For adults with overweight or obesity who don't have eating disorders, a wealth of studies show that regular and frequent weighing (daily or at least weekly) is associated with significantly greater weight reduction, and less weight regain over time.[3] One reason for this is that regular checking-in helps us notice if our weight is creeping up, so we can act quickly to get back where we want to be.

Weights or measures? I suggest using both. Use scales regularly to help understand how your body responds to things like the size of a meal, hydration levels, regularity of bowel movements and changes related to your menstrual cycle, so you can tell the difference between those changes and trends in your underlying weight. Use a tape measure for a more accurate way to track changes in body composition (fat vs. muscle).

---

[3] Some studies show that in adolescents and young adults (particularly females) with concerns about body shape, frequent self-weighing is associated with disordered eating, and is not recommended.

Weight

Weigh yourself in the morning when you get up. Do it naked, after urinating and before drinking.

Shape – track the tape

With the same tape measure you used earlier, measure:

Middle – using the same technique as for taking your baseline.

Natural waist – this is just above your belly button, and below your ribcage. It will probably be the narrowest part of your torso, but not necessarily.

Widest part – for most women this is likely to be across the top of your thighs and around your bottom. For men, it might be the same as the 'middle' measurement. Record exactly where you took the measurement, because this number is going to change over time!

Tops of your thighs – at the widest part before they meet your bottom. This is a useful place to measure if, like me, you tend to store more fat on your hips rather than your middle.

If you love data… measure other places too. Changes often show up in neck circumference, just above knees, and tops of the arms.

If your scales estimate fat content, note this as well. Changes in hydration affect this measurement, so for accurate comparison, always weigh first thing in the morning.

In the back of your journal or notebook, or on your computer, set up a table to record it all:

DATE	WEIGHT	MIDDLE	WAIST	WIDEST	THIGHS
Today					
This time next week					

Add extra columns if you want to keep other measurements

Once a week, write it down

My suggestion is to record weight and tape measurements every week until you reach your ideal weight. After that, measure fortnightly or so.

Because your weight will fluctuate a little day-to-day, there is nothing to be gained by recording a daily weight. This doesn't mean you can't weigh yourself every day if you want to – go right ahead! Daily weighing helps us become familiar with the subtle changes that occur at different times during the day, week or month. It can help us understand how much water we've been drinking, or how full our stomach is from our day's meals. But don't bother to record a daily weight.

Take photos

Photos of progress can be a strong motivator. Put on some undies that allow a good all-round view, and take two pictures – one from the front, the other side on. Once a month or so, take a new set of photos, wearing the same or similar clothing.

If one of your goals is to wear some favourite outfits again, try them on regularly to check how the fit is changing.

The first two kilos

When you first make a change in your eating habits, especially if you reduce carbohydrate intake, you might experience the sudden disappearance of 1–2 kg. If this happens, it will be due to what's often called 'water weight'. Once our body has used its easily available glucose for energy, it turns to its back-up stores of glucose – a substance called glycogen that's stored in our liver and muscles. Glycogen is 'attached' to water molecules, so when we use glycogen for energy, we excrete (as urine) the water it was attached to – about 2 kg worth.

We do need stores of glycogen, so our body rebuilds it straight away, next time we eat more carbs than we need for energy. This means that your weight may fluctuate over the first few weeks due to loss and gain of glycogen. Not something to worry about – the underlying steady downward trend in your measurements is from shedding body fat.

Mood and energy

Each week, spend a little time writing in your journal about how you're feeling – your mood and energy levels.

I know many people will struggle with this suggestion, as introspection of this sort is very personal. And you might have practical concerns that it won't be secure or private (*The secret diaries of…!*).

Becoming conscious of and familiar with the role that food and eating plays in your life will help change the way you eat, which is why I encourage using a journal. But you don't need to go the whole hog on this aspect if it makes you feel uncomfortable. Just make daily space in your head to think about these things.

Mood

Write down things that happened during the week to remind you of your goals, and of how important your healthy, vibrant body is.

Writing in a personal journal is often recommended as a way to improve well-being. While it's okay to record feelings of unhappiness, focus on speaking kindly to yourself, encouraging yourself, and always including things that made you feel happy or grateful.

Energy

In the beginning, a change in the way we eat can leave us feeling tired or listless. As our body gets used to these changes – different food, less sugar, smaller portions – we feel brighter, happier and more energetic.

If you're used to eating a lot of sugar or refined carbs, you may even feel unwell for the first two or three days. Take it as a sign that the millions of bacteria in your gut are adjusting to the change!

Think about your average energy level during the week and measure it on a scale ranging between 'extremely fatigued' and 'bursting with energy'. If you've been very up and down, an average energy level might not mean much. Instead, record how often during the week you felt exhausted, and how often you felt bright and ready for anything.

Maintaining your ideal weight – the two-kilo band

Old habits can creep back, particularly if you or your family have a history of overweight.

Once you reach your ideal weight, keep a regular watch on the scales, and take a weekly waist measurement. If your weight increases more than 2 kg, or waist measurement by 2 cm, it's time to check your eating habits, and return to the tactics in this book.

Gentle and prompt reminders to your body that its happiest weight is somewhere within a two-kilo band is much easier, and kinder, than allowing a larger increase that will be difficult to shift.

Are we there yet?

Real, safe and permanent reduction in body fat takes time. A realistic expectation is a change on the scales of about 2 kg, or up to 2 cm on your waist measurement, per month.

You might not see a clear trend for the first four weeks – but stick with it. Remember that you're building up a strong, stable core of eating behaviours, not changing everything overnight.

Exactly how much comes off will vary week to week, and it'll be affected by factors like how high your starting weight is compared with your target weight. The more you carry, the quicker it will probably leave, at least in the beginning. What your scales show will also be influenced by changes in muscle mass, so if you take up activities such as resistance training or weightlifting (excellent idea!), at first the changes might show up only in your waist measurements.

The state of your metabolism is also an important factor: if it's slow, especially as a result of years of restrictive dieting or inadequate protein, your body will be holding onto the extra weight. Chapter 7 has more on rehabilitating a sluggish metabolism.

Weight reduction won't be a steady, linear thing either. You might see nothing for a few weeks, then a real change, then another plateau. It could take months for your metabolism to return to a healthy state, allowing your weight to drop.

It helps to keep your eye on the overall goal – creating healthy eating habits. Remember that the most important thing is to make *lifelong changes in the way you eat*. Focus on practising and building these changes, not the speed at which you're seeing physical results.

HABIT HELPERS – MEASURING PROGRESS

Keep it regular. Weigh at least twice per week. Measure once a week, at the same time of day.

Keep records. If you really love data, set up an Excel spreadsheet and track a projected line of change, or do other fun things with your numbers.

Keep it up. Maintain a weekly weigh and measure, and record it, until you reach your target weight. After that, track your weight and measurements regularly (weekly or fortnightly). If the scales go up by more than 2 kg, or your largest measurement increases by more than 2 cm – it's time to pay more attention.

Be patient. Change will take time to show up.

Mindset matters: no blame, no shame. Tracking progress is only constructive if it's a positive reinforcement.

Weigh and measure with a curious, loving mind. No judgement.

REFLECTIONS

Treasure yourself

- What image will you create and keep in your head to remind you of your goals, and how important your healthy, vibrant body is? To symbolise '*I treasure my body*'?

- How might you describe the changes you'll make to your body composition? Will you lighten up, becoming lithe and free? Peel off the layers that weigh you down, that hide or smother you? Find your natural body shape?

Motivation matters

- Have you set your goals, checking that they're reasonable and motivated from a place of love?

Move it

Exercise is not the most significant part of reaching or keeping a healthy weight

Most of our weight is determined by what we put in our mouth, not by exercise (athletes aside). Only a small portion of our energy is used in deliberate exercise, varying between close to zero for a sedentary person, up to 10% for a highly active person exercising heavily every day.

Research indicates that unless we're doing significant amounts of vigorous exercise, we're unlikely to experience much weight or fat loss from exercise alone. It also shows that when we exercise more, we typically increase our food intake too, but don't reduce it when we exercise less. The bottom line from the research is that we can more effectively shed fat and prevent regain by eating better, rather than moving more (although ideally we'd do both!).

Exercise is important – it keeps our heart healthy, it keeps us flexible mentally and physically, and it helps keep us strong, just for starters. Muscles need fuel to function, so having good muscle mass keeps our metabolism moving, and this is essential for maintaining a healthy weight. Exercise has other important metabolic benefits too, helping to reduce systemic inflammation and increase insulin sensitivity. And, of course, exercise often helps motivate us to eat well.

But exercise isn't the *most important part* of reaching or keeping our ideal weight, and without also changing our eating habits, it will not bring us to a healthy weight.

We're built for moving – so move it!

Our bodies are designed to move – to be strong, fluid, fast, nimble. Moving is joyful.

Ride a bike because you love the cool wind in your face. The exhilaration of hurtling down a hill.

Lift weights because you love the challenge. Because it means you can wrangle your children, your dog, or your partner.

Run because you love the air filling your lungs, the sense of your legs moving, precise and strong.

Walk because you love to be in nature, contemplative and alone inside your own head, with your own thoughts. Or with friends, enjoying their communion.

Practise yoga because you love the quiet stillness that comes with breathing deeply into a pose.

As your new eating habits bring changes to your body shape, exercise will become an even more joyful motivator, as you find yourself with more energy and mobility.

Keep doing whatever physical activity you enjoy. If you're not doing anything, find some form of movement that you enjoy – and this is just as important for people with mobility restrictions as it is for those without. Do it because it keeps you positive, strong and flexible, and motivated to look after yourself. Aim for at least 20 minutes a day, every day.

Exercise is not punishment or compensation for eating 'too much', or 'the wrong stuff'. It's not an excuse to do those things either.

Lift heavy things

Building up muscle mass increases our metabolic rate, helping us reach and maintain a healthy weight.

You don't need to join a gym or buy a set of weights, although if that's what you enjoy, go your hardest. Muscle mass is built by resistance training. There are many ways to do it, including with free weights and by lifting your own body weight, for instance through many yoga poses, push ups, squats, lunges and skipping. Make the most of everyday opportunities to lift and carry, too – shopping, children, gardening and while doing household chores.

Lifting weights also protects bone density. This is especially important for women, particularly as we get older, during and after menopause.

...and stand up straight

While we're on the physical side of things – stand (and sit) up straight! Poor posture and abdominal muscle tone affect our digestion, making it more difficult for food to move through our system, potentially leading to constipation, bloating and a pot-belly. Good posture improves energy levels and increases muscle strength, especially in your core and back, which in turn help maintain a higher metabolism.

Pull your belly button towards your spine, slide your shoulder blades down your back, and tuck in your tailbone just a little. Now look in the mirror. You're strong; powerful. You own your body; it carries you proudly through life. Feel the confidence and embrace it.

Keep feeling your belly muscles supporting you as you go about your daily life, including as you sit at a desk. As your stomach and shoulder muscles grow stronger, you'll be able to hold a better posture without even thinking about it. This simple habit will also do your neck, shoulders and back a favour.

What about 'calories in – calories out'?

A calorie is a unit of energy – specifically in this context, the amount of energy (fuel for our body) provided by an item of food.[4] For example, two medium eggs give us around 155 calories.

We're frequently told that you 'will' shed the kilos if you simply obey the equation *calories out exceed calories in*. That is, if you exercise enough to use up all the energy you eat, everything will be fine.

In theory, this might sound logical. But in practice, it doesn't stack up, for a number of reasons:

Our estimates are wrong. We are wildly out in our estimates on both sides of the equation: the energy value of what we eat (and how quickly we store any excess energy as fat), and the energy value of the exercise we do. Quite simply – there isn't enough time in the day to exercise sufficiently to make up for poor eating habits.

We get hungry and tired. Simply reducing calories to shed weight leaves us feeling tired, hungry and despondent *unless we're choosing the right sort of food*. Exactly the opposite of how we should be feeling. This book is all about changing eating habits (what, why and how) so that it's easy to choose the food that keeps you feeling satisfied and energetic.

We eat at the wrong times. We commonly eat large meals far too late in the day. Eating in time with our body's natural body clock (circadian rhythm), so that we *eat breakfast every morning, and finish eating well before we head for bed*, results in a higher metabolism, greater fat burning and reduced fat storage than the identical quantity of calories eaten at the 'wrong' time. The next chapter has more about eating at the right time.

---

[4] Another unit to measure food energy is the kilojoule (kJ) – there are about 4.2 kJ to a calorie. This book uses calories only.

We each have different metabolic rates, which are altered by the 'what, when and how' of eating. Metabolic rate (the 'calories out' side of the equation) varies widely between individuals and is altered by what, when, how, how much and how often we eat, and also by our own unique gut microbiome. For example, extremely low-calorie diets reduce our metabolic rate, and keep it down. High-protein diets increase it. Chapter 7 has more on both maintaining metabolic rate and the importance of our microbiome.

It doesn't account for metabolic disorders caused by high sugar intake, or by highly processed foods. High intake of refined grains (flour), sugar and processed foods significantly increases the risk of diseases such as fatty liver, and metabolic disorders such as insulin resistance, which in turn cause weight gain. Chapter 4 has more detail on sugar and processed food.

Different foods use different amounts of energy to digest. Protein, for example, uses much more energy to digest than sugar, starch or fat – so a high-protein diet increases the 'calories out' side of the equation by raising our metabolic rate more than other types of diets.

Different foods are metabolised differently, and have different long-term health effects. Eating 100 calories worth of cake has a vastly different effect on our body than eating 100 calories of green vegetables. Different types of food use different metabolic pathways for digestion, and vary in their vitamin and mineral content as well as their effect on our gut health.

It's true that to shed body fat, we need to eat less. *But just as importantly*, we need to eat the right things, at the right time, and in the right way, without feeling hungry or deprived. Five for Life shows how to do that.

HABIT HELPERS – MOVE IT

Take twenty. Spend at least 20 minutes a day in energetic movement – try dancing, yoga, walking or gardening. Do what you love.

Think differently about how you use your body. Every day, look for opportunities to use your body. Take the stairs, or park a little further away. Carry your baby or child on your back or front instead of using a pram or pusher. Focus on your core as you move – whether it's walking between offices, housework, gardening, or getting in and out of the car.

Stand tall, be proud. Posture matters. Stand and sit up straight; pull in your belly button.

Don't lie down if you can sit, don't sit if you can stand, don't stand if you can walk.[5]

REFLECTIONS

- What do you do every day to keep your body moving?
- Why do you do it?
- What do you love about it?

---

[5]   Winston Churchill (Prime Minister of Britain during the Second World War) said, 'Economy of effort. Never stand up when you can sit down, and never sit down when you can lie down.' He was not a healthy weight. If you want to be a healthy weight – use your body in the best way you can. It's what it was designed for.

Manage stress and get enough sleep

Stress and poor sleep are potent causes of excess weight, and a common outcome of neglecting to treasure our own selves.

There's a lot to say about both of these, so they have dedicated sections in Chapter 8. For now, the short story is this:

- Unmanaged, chronic stress keeps the primary stress hormone, cortisol, at constantly high levels in our blood. Chronically high cortisol increases our appetite – and especially our appetite for the type of food that will make us fat: sugar and other processed food. Cortisol also affects *where we store fat* – increasing the dangerous visceral fat deposits deep in our belly, around and inside our organs.

- Poor sleep patterns disrupt our hormones and interfere with our circadian rhythm. Lack of quality sleep increases our desire for unhealthful food.

HABIT HELPERS – STRESS AND SLEEP

Chill out. To help reduce weight permanently, manage stress effectively and improve your sleep. There's lots more about this in Chapter 8.

Recap – Treasure your body

Totally you. You are a whole and multi-faceted human being, and you are not your appearance.

Loving you. Looking after your precious body is an act of love. Each time you eat and drink is an opportunity to remember this and make it real.

Committing to you. Practise the pillars of healthy eating in some way, every day. Write down your commitment and remind yourself of it first thing every morning, and during the day.

Build your team. Hang around people who whole-heartedly support you.

Be patient, not perfect. It's okay to get things right 80% of the time. Don't fret the 20%.

CHAPTER THREE

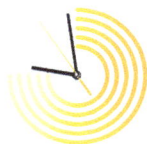

WHEN TO EAT

To reach and stay at your ideal weight, it's essential to eat at the right time. This means two things:

1. Eat when you're *hungry.*

2. Eat in sync with your *circadian rhythm.*

In this chapter, we'll talk about:

- understanding why you eat. Recognise hunger and be aware of the other reasons why you eat. Resist deep-seated habits and peer pressure for eating when you aren't hungry

- recognising when it's time to stop eating. Reduce portion sizes to stop overstretching your stomach and retrain the way it sends the 'enough' message to your brain

- eating regularly to support healthy eating habits and your own metabolism

- eating at the right clock time for your body. Find out about the circadian rhythm and why it's so essential to *eat early* – starting with breakfast and ending with a small and early evening meal

- following the *Five for Life Fast* described in the last section of this chapter, for a practical and effective way to do time-restricted eating.

Eating at the right time – the short story

Eat when you're hungry. Stop when you're not.

Identifying and understanding what triggers our eating is the first part of the 'when' of eating.

Recognise hunger – We eat for many reasons, and hunger often isn't one of them. Eating when we don't need to takes us further from our weight goals. Ask yourself – *if I'm not hungry, and it isn't my regular mealtime, why should I eat this?* Make a choice that supports your faithful body.

Recognise satiety – Satiety is the sense that we've had enough to eat, and that we're no longer hungry. Eating slowly and attentively helps us notice when we've had enough.

Eat smaller portions – Eating smaller portions helps stop over-eating. It also prevents our stomach from overstretching, allowing our body to re-learn the signal for when it's had enough to eat.

Eat regularly – People who eat regularly tend to have more stable blood sugar, lower body fat and better appetite control than those who eat irregularly or skip meals. Eat like a lean person – eat regularly.

Eat in sync with your circadian rhythm

The second part of the 'when' of eating is about watching the clock, and it matters more than you'd expect.

When we eat, in relation to our internal body clock (circadian rhythm), has a significant impact on our weight and how much fat we carry. Disrupting our circadian rhythm – including by eating at the wrong time – not only causes weight gain, but also contributes to metabolic diseases and is associated with other illnesses.

To support your circadian rhythm to shed excess fat and keep it off – eat early, and follow these four steps:

- *Eat breakfast.* Eat breakfast every day for improved weight and body composition, for metabolic health, and for mental focus.

- *Eat most before 3 pm.* Having the majority of our energy intake in the earlier part of the day helps reduce weight. The later we eat, the more likely we are to store those calories as fat.

- *Eat least in the evening.* Have your last meal early, and make it light.

- *…Then stop.* Don't have any calories after your last meal.

If you want to do intermittent fasting, try the *Five for Life Fast* set out at the end of the chapter.

Understanding why you eat

Why do we eat?

Why do we eat? Why do *you, personally,* eat? It's an interesting question.

Most Australians are now over-fed, so we seldom eat because we're hungry. There are all sorts of motivations for eating, and it's an important reason why so many of us carry unhealthy amounts of weight. *We eat when we aren't hungry.*

Recognise and acknowledge what triggers your eating, and if it isn't bringing you closer to your ideal weight, it's time to substitute for new habits.

Out of boredom or worry

We might wander to the kitchen or pantry out of boredom or as a form of procrastination (this is me!). We feel in need of something, and not being sure what it is, look for something to put in our mouths.

Many of us also eat when we're worried or stressed. Reaching for sugar is an especially common response to being upset, as sugar gives us a short 'high', which can relieve anxiety, even if just for a few minutes. But once the high is over, we crave another – and therefore more sugar.

Desire! We like it, or want it

We often eat just because we like the taste of a food, or even crave it. How many times have you eaten something just because the thought or sight of it triggered a strong sense of desire?

Our sense of sight and smell are closely associated with our expectations of reward – the sight of a brightly iced, glossy donut, the smell of bread straight from the oven. For many of us it's almost irresistible – this is sometimes referred to as 'hedonic hunger', and it's associated with *certain types of food*. Chapter 4 looks at how to identify and avoid those foods.

To be social

Food is essential for life and health, and this makes the preparation and sharing of food a strong symbol of love and friendship. Eating with friends or family is a way to share time together in one place, in a nurturing atmosphere.

From peer pressure

You might call this the dark side of social eating.

Have you ever been around people who are themselves an unhealthy weight, who want you to join them eating? Do they say things like 'just one won't hurt', 'you can diet tomorrow', 'you could eat anything you want, with a figure like yours', or 'you're looking too scrawny'? Consider what might be motivating their comments, and let your own sense of wellness and care for your body guide you.

It's incredibly empowering to sometimes just say 'no thanks'. It's also a self-reinforcing habit.

Because it's 'time'

It's lunchtime, or dinnertime, or breakfast time. We learn this habit from a very early age. One reason for learning it – and also for keeping it – is convenience. Households tend to function more smoothly when everyone eats their main meals together. If your workplace has set break times, you might have little say over when you eat.

But there's more to it than convenience: eating regularly also helps us reach and stay at a healthy weight (more on this later).

Identify eating triggers and make a conscious choice

Some of the reasons we eat are healthy – for our body and spirit. Others are not healthy at all.

To nurture new habits, it's vital to identify clearly, each time we eat, *why* we're eating. To make conscious choices about eating, and to enjoy food in a way that supports our whole selves.

Eat when you're hungry, stop when you're not

Recognise hunger

Feeling hungry is our body's natural signal to eat, and we should eat when we feel the beginning of that signal. However, most of us eat so frequently it might be difficult to remember the last time we felt truly hungry. Time to practise recognising hunger. It's not dangerous, I promise!

We all experience hunger a bit differently, but it's usually an empty, rumbling stomach sensation, and may come with irritability, loss of focus or a headache.

It takes up to four hours for food to pass through our stomach completely after eating, so one way to practise hunger is to delay eating for four to five hours after a meal. By this time, your stomach will be empty, and the sensation you feel is likely to be hunger. Another way is to stop eating around five hours before bed. You may wake during the night feeling hungry, and you will probably wake in the morning feeling hungry.

Eating regular, small meals helps train our body to feel hunger at the right time. The right time is in time with our internal body clock – our circadian rhythm. More on that later in this chapter.

Hunger and the overstretched stomach

Regularly overeating makes our stomach stretchier, so it can hold more food. This increased stretchiness (distensibility) changes the way our brain understands 'hunger' and 'fullness'. When we regularly overeat, our stomach becomes used to feeling full, and won't send the 'enough' signal to the brain until we've already had 'too much'. Like a balloon that has been filled and released many times, it will be constantly looking for a little bit more before it feels full. It will also feel empty more quickly, sending us in search of a top-up.

Over time, overeating becomes the norm for our stomach and brain.

Craving vs. hunger

It's easy to mistake craving for hunger, especially if you're not used to recognising true hunger. When you first feel a craving for food outside of a regular meal or snack time, drink a couple of glasses of water, then wait for half an hour or so. If you still feel a need for food, bring forward your next planned meal or snack. I'm not suggesting this approach fixes cravings (if only!) but it will help consciously pinpoint the difference between hunger and craving. Cravings are a serious burden for many people, and Chapter 10 has more about them.

Stop eating when you've had enough – recognise satiety

It's logical that if we only eat when we're hungry, we'll stop eating when we've had enough. But this often doesn't happen, and we just keep eating.

Learn to notice when you've had 'just enough' and recognise it as the signal to stop eating. One method that can help is stopping partway through the meal. Put your cutlery down. Look up from your plate, and consciously become aware of your body's sensations.

When food is very dense in calories, such as high-fat or high-sugar food, it's easy to eat a lot of it quickly before we feel a sense of fullness. Be aware that energy-dense food can escape your 'off' switch, and pay extra attention.

> ### Knowing when you've had enough – Hara hachi bun me
>
> The Japanese islands of Okinawa are home to the world's largest concentration of healthy people aged 100 or over.[6] Okinawan elders typically have a BMI of 18–22, which is the lower end of the healthy BMI range.
>
> Okinawans say the phrase *'hara hachi bun me'* before each meal. It roughly means 'eat until 80% full'.

Let go of fear

Many of us still live with an innate scarcity mindset that can unconsciously drive overeating. Relax. If you're still hungry when you've finished, there's nothing preventing you from having more.

---

[6] Okinawa is one of the so-called 'Blue Zones' – a place in the world where people live remarkably long, healthy lives.

Putting it into practice

There are plenty of challenges to the habit of *eating when you're hungry (and not when you're not)*, especially in early days of change. The second breakfast, the mid-afternoon slump-busting snack, the after-exercise 'treat', the office morning tea or birthday cake.

And waiting to derail 'stop when you're 80% full' are things like peer pressure when you're eating out with friends, finishing food on your children's plates, and being used to always eating what's put in front of you.

Understanding about **portion sizes**, and the importance of **eating regularly**, are two things that will help – they're discussed in the next couple of sections. **Eating mindfully**, which is the focus of Chapter 6, is also a helpful practice. Chapter 10 includes practical suggestions for tackling everyday challenges.

HABIT HELPERS – EAT WHEN YOU'RE HUNGRY, STOP WHEN YOU'RE NOT

Ask first. If it's not your regular mealtime, and you're tempted to eat, ask yourself *'Am I hungry?'* Remind yourself what hunger feels like for you. Drink water if you're not sure, and ask again a bit later.

Commit to it. Begin each meal with a conscious commitment to stop eating when you're no longer hungry. Have a short phrase to say to yourself (even *hara hachi bun me*, if you can happily get your tongue around it).

Take it slowly. Chew slowly and thoroughly, so you notice when you've had enough. Check in on your sensations while you're eating. It's a fact that people who eat slowly tend to be leaner than those who eat quickly. (More about this in Chapter 6.)

> ***Enjoy it.*** Welcome the physical sensation of having eaten just the right amount. No longer hungry, but not full or uncomfortable.
>
> ***Say it.*** *'I'll let my digestive system rest until my next meal.'*

REFLECTIONS

Reasons why you eat

- Understand why you eat, recognising triggers other than hunger. Write them down.

- Identify the triggers you find most troublesome – in what circumstances are you most likely to eat when you aren't hungry? Or to eat until you're over-full? Or to reach for products you know won't help you shed excess weight?

Stop eating when you've had enough

- Do you often keep eating when you're full? Can you put your finger on why?

Eat the right amount

Most of us eat too much.

There are many reasons, but an important one is that in Australia and most of the Western world, our portion sizes are typically too big. Each time we eat a meal or snack, it's often too much. Over the day, this adds up to '*far too much*'.

Portion creep

It's not our imagination – research shows that the larger our portions, the more we tend to eat. And we don't reduce the size of our next meal to compensate for overeating at the previous meal.

We've become used to seeing and expecting large portions of food in shops, restaurants and fast-food outlets. Being surrounded by this oversized visual diet drives our perception of what is the 'right' amount to eat. It's probably also led to a habit of serving large portions at home.

Push back and create a new feedback loop

With conscious practice, we can effectively replace a habit of expecting, serving and eating larger portions. We're unlikely to stop *seeing* extra-large serves any time soon, because food manufacturers continue to target us with crafty advertisements. But with awareness, we can push back and create our own healthy habits around portion size.

Reducing food portions, both at home and when we're out, can help us feel very differently about what is a 'normal' and appropriate portion size. Studies show that just as we don't compensate for a large meal by having a small one next time, the same goes for switching to small meals. When we eat a small meal, we don't generally 'make up for it' by eating more at the next meal – studies show we're just as likely to eat a small portion again. The end result? If we reduce portion sizes, we're likely to eat less overall. In time, our stomach will also learn to signal earlier to our brain that it's had enough, so we feel fuller on smaller portions. A supportive feedback loop.

What is the right amount?

If you've been used to having oversized meals, it will feel strange at first to adjust. It will also look very different on your plate from what you're used to.

The 'right' portion size varies depending on what you're eating. High-fibre bulky foods (a pile of dry-fried greens, or a leafy summer salad) take up more space than dense food like a piece of chicken or steak, avocado or nuts.

You might be familiar with the idea of using your hand to help decide portion size. It works well because our hands are generally in proportion to our height and overall frame.

As I'm advocating small, frequent meals, an appropriate portion is roughly:

- Protein: Fish, meat or poultry – a piece the size and thickness of your palm. Pulses or tofu – an amount the size of your fist.

- Non-starchy vegetables: One loose fist of cooked vegetables, or two of raw vegetables. *Beware dressings on vegetables and salads* unless you made them yourself. Commercial dressings can add considerable extra sugar and processed vegetable oil, both of which contribute to weight gain.

- Fat: One 10 g serve of fat. There may be enough fat in your protein serve (e.g. a 100 g piece of salmon has about 15 g fat), but if not, add some. Cold-pressed olive, avocado or nut oil (about half a tablespoon), raw nuts or seeds (a tablespoon) or half an avocado each have about 10 g fat, and are good choices. Make sure you count fat used in cooking, or in salad or vegetable dressings.

- Carbs: Grains and starchy vegetables (quinoa, spelt, wholegrain pasta, wholegrain bread, brown rice, potato or sweet potato) or fruit are high-quality choices. At most, have as much as would fit in your cupped hand, *in total*. If your meal's protein source is pulses, reduce or omit extra carbs. You ***don't need to add carb foods to every meal***.

If the meal is 'meat/tofu and veg', it's easy to use this method. If it's a mix, such as stir-fry, casserole, or curry, it is trickier to estimate ingredients and identify which part is the protein source, and where the carbs are. You'll get better at it over time.

A simpler way is to aim for a total meal size that's approximately equivalent to one large fist of mostly protein and a little fat, then add your non-starchy vegetables, with a small amount of grains or starchy vegetables *if required*. At least half your plate should be non-starchy vegetables, and about one third should be a source of protein.

Chapter 4 has all the detail on protein, fat and carbs.

> ### Plate sizes
>
> Years ago, we bought a new dishwasher and discovered that our dinner plates were too large for it. Rather than buy a new set, we began to use cereal bowls for everyday meals instead. The dishwasher could hold more of them in a load, they were easier for young children to carry and hold… and so we just got into the habit.
>
> Apart from convenience, the other thing about cereal bowls is that they don't hold that much, and it's meant that, unintentionally, our evening meals have been relatively small. Still are, because although we did eventually buy new plates, the cereal bowl habit has stuck!

Eating out

Awareness is critical. Be aware that portions served in restaurants, cafes and fast-food outlets are too big. Decide to eat only an appropriate portion – about a fistful, plus non-starchy vegetables. Vegetables are usually prepared with dressings and sauces that add significant extra carbs and calories. If the vegetables can be prepared dressing-free, that's great; otherwise, limit vegetables too.

Chapter 10 has specific tips on eating out (including taking leftovers home).

No contest!

Smaller adults need less energy (fewer calories) than larger adults, and less than growing children. If you need fewer calories than others in your household, or people you eat with at work or socially, accept that you won't be matching them for meal size. In an eating-out setting, this is even more important. Serving sizes don't arrive at the table 'tailor-made' for our own size and needs. It's a one-size-fits-all arrangement, even if that's going to take us to a size we don't want to be.

Eating what's put in front of you

Your parents, or someone else important in your upbringing, might have told you to 'eat what's put in front of you'. They might have meant *'don't complain about what I've cooked for you – that's it'*, or *'eat everything on your plate'* – or both.

If this was said to you, your *eat-everything-on-the-plate* habit might be deeply ingrained. And it will get seriously in the way of portion control.

Time to change. The best way to start is by acknowledging that this message has seeped into your psyche. But it doesn't control you. There are two practical ways to tackle it:

- *Serve your own food.* If someone else is serving, practise saying *'just a small bit for me, thanks'*.
- *Learn to leave it.* Think of leftovers as a gift for the following day – a meal or snack that's ready-to-go, no need for extra food prep time.

Are you overstretched?

Everyone's stomach when it's empty, no matter their adult size and weight, is about 25 cm long, and would hold less than ½ cup (100 ml). But our stomachs are 'distensible' and can comfortably contain about one litre of chewed food or liquid. If stuffed full, a stomach can hold up to four litres.

The more frequently we fill our stomach with a large meal, the happier it will be to stretch to accommodate more. A stomach that is used to being overfilled tells the brain it wants more, even when we don't need the extra nutrients.

The good news is that eating smaller portions reduces our stomach's stretchiness and changes the way it signals our brain that it's full. Best of all, it doesn't take long. When we stop overfilling our stomach, it gets used to feeling full on smaller amounts of food, reducing distensibility over three to four weeks.

In the beginning...

Your stomach *will probably complain* when you first move to smaller portions. If it's used to being overfilled, that's the signal it's looking for to register 'enough'. Welcome this complaint, because it's a sign that you're moving in the right direction to re-tune your brain-gut connection.

Retrain your stomach gradually by eating smaller portions – just enough to stop the grumble, not to fill up.

Are you eating *enough*?

While most of us eat too much, some of us don't – and are still overweight.

Periodic dieting with severe calorie restriction makes it difficult to shed fat and increases the likelihood that we'll just get fatter. Our resting metabolism accounts for up to 80% of the 'energy out' side of the weight equation, so if our energy intake is too low (cutting daily calories below about 1,200 for days or weeks on end), *especially if we're skimping on protein or fat*, our body thinks there's a famine on and reduces its resting metabolic rate to compensate. It also increases the amount of body fat it stores, to keep itself safe from the possibility of another famine, some time in the future.

What's the remedy? The answer to permanent and safe weight reduction is to encourage our body to voluntarily relinquish excess body fat. Return to *small, regular and frequent meals of the right sort of food* in sufficient quantities, as described in Chapter 4. You can get your metabolic rate back on track, but it may take a little while.

HABIT HELPERS – PORTION CAUTION

Scale it down – use smaller crockery and cutlery. Studies show a small but significant decrease in energy intake from using smaller tools. When you're eating at home, serve your meals on smaller crockery – e.g. a shallow cereal bowl instead of a dinner plate. Use smaller cutlery – a dessert fork and bread-and-butter knife. Or children's cutlery if you have it.

Always put your food on a plate. Never eat from boxes or bags. It's too difficult to properly judge the quantity, and you also miss out on the visual cue for mentally registering the meal, which is part of what helps our brain understand when it has had enough.

Divide and conquer! Eating out? Share it, leave it, or take it away. If you're at home and used to serving a larger portion at lunch or dinner – divide it into thirds. Two thirds now, one third for a meal or snack tomorrow.

Last is least. The closer it is to bedtime, the smaller your meal should be.

Think it; say it. '*Overstretching makes me sick.*'

REFLECTIONS

- What meals or snacks do you find most difficult in terms of managing serving size? Is it restaurant meals, or food prepared with love by family or friends? Or highly salted or sweet items?

- What tactics will you use to manage portion sizes?

Eat regularly

Keep it regular

Some of us stay at a healthy weight on three meals plus a couple of snacks, while others do well on only two meals per day. Although the best meal frequency may vary between people, studies show that the overall *regularity* of meals is very important.

The evidence is clear that for most of us, and especially those who have difficulty maintaining a healthy weight, small, regular meals guard against excess weight gain and metabolic syndrome. Eating the right food regularly:

- helps keep blood sugar stable and helps prevent excess hunger during the day
- results in lower energy intake overall
- reduces the chance of seeking poor-quality, high-calorie foods at the next meal.

If you tend to have little appetite during the day, or at breakfast time, starting a regular food routine will help develop healthier eating habits.

What about frequency?

Does it matter how *many* meals we have each day? Most large population-based studies show that eating frequently is associated with lower risk of obesity, diabetes and heart disease. Based on this evidence, the American Heart Association has issued a statement that frequent meals should be preferred.[7] On the other hand, other analyses conclude that the regularity of eating, the timing of eating, and the macronutrient balance (proportion of protein, fat and carbs) are just as important as meal frequency.[8]

---

[7]   St-Onge (2017) Meal timing and frequency: implications for cardiovascular disease prevention: a scientific statement from the American Heart Association.

[8]   Paoli (2019) The influence of meal frequency and timing on health in humans: the role of fasting.

For people who have no difficulty maintaining their happy weight with regular but infrequent meals, there's no reason to change. But if you're aiming to reduce weight, the evidence favours eating at least three meals per day, *including breakfast*. People who eat three or more meals per day tend to have lower body fat and better appetite control, while eating *fewer* than three meals is linked to increases in body fat, including visceral fat.

Advocates of eating just once or twice a day, and especially skipping breakfast, claim that the body needs to go into 'fasting' mode in order to burn fat. That much is true! However, we also now know a lot more about the importance of our circadian rhythm and its impact on our weight. The next two sections have more on the circadian rhythm and fasting, and introduce the ***Five for Life Fast***, an easy-to-follow form of intermittent fasting that supports our circadian rhythm.

If we want to increase our fast by shortening the daytime 'eating window', but at the same time don't want to eat meals that are too large, or risk getting excessively hungry and reaching for the nearest high-carb danger zone food, it makes sense to eat small, nutritious meals frequently. So: improve your chances of safe and permanent weight reduction by having regular, small and high-protein meals, starting with breakfast and fitting all nutrients into an eating window that ends by about 6 pm. If you need to eat later than that, make it a token meal only.

HABIT HELPERS – EAT REGULARLY

Routine regime. Decide when you'll eat (at least three times per day) and stick to it. It's easier to establish a new habit if you make a conscious pledge that removes other options.

Plan it out. Decide what to eat! Plan ahead for the day. It's easy to reach for the right food when it's already prepared, or you know what you're having. On the other hand, not being ready for mealtimes can easily derail our intentions.

> ***Mere morsels.*** Eating frequently means that some of your meals might be quite small. Chapters 10 and 11 have some tips on healthy snacking and smaller meals. There are more ideas in Appendix A and on the Five for Life website.

The circadian sync (*burn fat while you sleep!*)

Our circadian rhythm is our own internal body clock. It plays a crucial role in our body's systems, including hormone production and metabolism, cell regeneration and body temperature, which all change during the 24-hour cycle.

Disrupting this rhythm is bad for our sleep, and detrimental to our physical and mental health. In particular, eating at the wrong time for our body clock contributes to excess fat storage and metabolic diseases. For most of us, the wrong time to eat is night-time.

Just as disrupting our circadian rhythm can lead to overweight or obesity, eating in sync with it helps to shed fat, and keep it off. It's literally a case of 'burn fat while you sleep'. But this won't happen if your body has to deal with a heap of carbs or alcohol (or both) before it gets to the fat.

The short story – eat early

Ever heard the saying '*Eat like a king in the morning, a prince at noon, and a peasant at dinner*'? It's old (the thoughts of a twelfth-century philosopher named Maimonides), but pretty close to the mark, and matches what we know about eating in time with our circadian rhythm.

Numerous studies confirm the importance of eating early to maintain lower body fat, as well as good metabolic and heart health. Among these are studies following tens of thousands of people over many years, showing that those who often skip breakfast or lunch are more likely to be overweight and have heart disease, compared with those who consistently eat breakfast. The reasons why this is the case aren't yet fully established, but it's clear that we burn more fat over a 24-hour period if we eat most of our calories during the first part of the day, while food we eat later is more likely to be stored as fat. Studies also show that most people's bodies burn more carbs more effectively in the morning than in the afternoon. And they also show that if we eat breakfast, we burn significantly more energy overall during the first part of the day.

This doesn't mean that everyone who eats early, rather than late, will easily keep their weight where they want it, but the evidence is that *eating early significantly improves your odds*.

Eating early – some recent studies

In the first major controlled study of the effects of early eating, two groups ate the same amount and type of food for three months. The food plans were high in protein and low in carbs. One group had their largest meal in the morning and smallest at night; the other group did the opposite. Those who ate most in the morning and least at night shed *more than twice as much weight*, and *reduced their waist measurements by twice as much* as the group who ate most in the evening. Fat levels in the blood of the 'early' eaters decreased by 33%, but in the 'late' eaters, it increased by 14%.[9]

In a 2020 trial, two groups ate exactly the same food over a 56-hour period, while they remained inside individual calorimetric chambers that measured their precise energy expenditure. One group ate at 8 am and had their last meal at 5.45 pm. The other group started at 12.30 pm and had their last meal at 10 pm. Both groups fasted for 14 hours each night – the only difference was that the breakfast-eating

---

[9] Jakubowicz (2013) High caloric intake at breakfast vs. dinner differentially influences weight loss of overweight and obese women.

group fasted from 6 pm until breakfast the next day, while the breakfast-skipping group fasted from 10.30 pm until lunchtime the following day.

The breakfast-eating group metabolised significantly more fat while they slept, and throughout the whole period, than the breakfast-skipping, late diners.[10]

Eating early in the Blue Zone

Residents of so-called 'Blue Zones' (locations where people average the longest and healthiest lives) eat their biggest meal, and most of their daily energy intake, during the first half of the day. They have their smallest meal in the late afternoon or early evening, and are typically very lean.[11]

The circadian sync: four simple steps

Eating in time with your circadian rhythm means following *four simple steps*:

1. Eat breakfast.

2. Have most of your fuel before 3 pm.

3. Have your evening meal early (at least three or four hours before bed).

4. Then stop. Don't eat after that.

---

[10] Kelly (2020) Eating breakfast and avoiding late-evening snacking sustains lipid oxidation.

[11] The term 'Blue Zone' is owned by Dan Buettner, who wrote the book *The Blue Zones: 9 lessons for living longer from the people who've lived the longest.* The five originally studied Blue Zones were Okinawa in Japan, Sardinia in Italy, Nicoya in Costa Rica, Icaria in Greece, and the Seventh Day Adventist community in Loma Linda, California.

Eat breakfast

It's true – eat breakfast. Don't skip it. Have a nourishing breakfast that's high in protein and fibre.

Eating breakfast is important for maintaining healthy weight and body fat, and for keeping us metabolically healthy: the right levels of blood sugar, blood lipids (fats and cholesterol), blood pressure and waist circumference. Numerous studies following thousands of people over many years consistently show the strong link between breakfast-eating and reduced risk of overweight and obesity, type 2 diabetes and cardiovascular disease. Quality randomised controlled trials indicate that the reason for this strong correlation is likely to be that eating breakfast results in lower total cholesterol and LDL:HDL cholesterol ratio, lower blood sugar and better insulin response after meals, compared with skipping breakfast.

Skipping breakfast in the name of intermittent fasting

Skipping breakfast so that the daytime eating window is shorter (e.g. from noon until 8 pm) is popular right now, possibly because the evidence that time-restricted eating by fasting for 14 hours overnight is good, has got mixed up with the idea that it's healthy to do this by skipping breakfast – which for most people, it isn't. You might also have heard the myth that *'breakfast was invented by an American man named Kellogg'*. Sounds catchy, but it's not true, although no doubt Kellogg was a keen advocate of cereal for breakfast.

Studies are clear that reducing eating hours will probably help you shed weight, but this may simply be because a smaller eating window leads to lower energy intake overall. A series of carefully controlled studies since about 2013 show that 'late' eating windows are associated with adverse metabolic health markers such as higher blood glucose and lower insulin sensitivity, and may also result in loss of more lean body mass than body fat. Late fasting is also contrary to what we know about the well-studied benefits of eating most of our fuel earlier in the day.

While we probably all know someone who shed excess fat by skipping breakfast, or perhaps it's worked for you previously, the evidence is against this being successful for many people, especially in the longer term. If the skipped breakfast was toast, cereal and fruit juice, there would be some benefit just from removing these low-quality carbs from the diet. But if, over time, carbs and other sources of energy are added back later in the day, weight and body fat will be regained.

If you want the best chance of reducing body fat and improving your metabolic health and mental focus – eat breakfast. The *Five for Life Fast* described later in this chapter shows how to marry breakfast with intermittent fasting.

What does a best breakfast look like?

Breakfast is a meal eaten within one to two hours of rising.

Research shows that breakfast **high in protein and fibre** helps us feel full for longer, and decreases blood sugar spikes. A good breakfast also has a medium amount of healthy fat (e.g. from eggs, avocado, nuts or seeds), and may include some high-quality carbs (e.g. from milk or yoghurt, or wholegrain bread).[12]

A good breakfast has no sugar or low-quality, starchy carbs. So that means no flavoured yoghurt or milk, no processed cereal, no fruit juice, and limited toast (wholegrain only).

Here are some breakfast suggestions – you can find more on the Five for Life website too.

Eggs! Two poached, boiled, scrambled or fried eggs make an excellent breakfast, with unlimited steamed kale or other greens and a small handful of nuts. If you like, have them with a single piece of toast, from high-quality bread.

---

[12] Chapter 4 has more on protein, fat and carbs and why our body needs them. It includes a Traffic Light Table with examples of high-quality protein, fats and carbs.

Easy poached eggs

Half fill a small saucepan with boiling water. Add ¼ cup plain white vinegar – just the ordinary, home-brand vinegar. Nothing fancy, or the eggs will look and taste quite strange. Bring the water back to a gentle boil.

Break an egg and slide it into the boiling water. Then add the other one. Turn the heat down to simmer for four or five minutes, depending how firm you like your eggs. Lift them out now and then with a slotted spoon and poke the yolk to test.

The best bread

High-quality bread is heavy, dense, and made with whole grains. Preferably, it's sourdough.

'Wholegrain bread' doesn't mean white bread that's got bits of whole grains scattered through it, that get caught in your teeth and, if you're unlucky, in crevices inside your intestines.

Wholegrain means that the flour has been ground from whole grains: it includes all parts of the grain, including the nutritious germ and the bran. Wholegrain bread will state this on its label, or if you're buying from a bakery, ask the baker. Look for bread that includes some grains other than wheat – spelt is a good one.

Wholegrain sourdough bread is more expensive than refined-flour bread, but you'll be eating much less of it.

Plain yoghurt. A cup of plain unsweetened yoghurt with some raw nuts, berries and rolled oats scattered through it makes *part* of a good breakfast, but you'll need to add an extra protein source to make a full meal.

Not fruit yoghurt, not vanilla flavoured… just plain. Greek, low fat, high protein, pot set, or biodynamic – whichever you prefer, provided it's plain. If you're used to sweet food, it may take your tastebuds a little while to adjust to the tart, creamy flavour.

Use non-dairy yoghurts (e.g. coconut or soy) with care, and check the nutrition label. They frequently have added sugars and other ingredients (even in the plain varieties) and are often lower in protein than their dairy counterparts.

Fish. Have some smoked salmon in your omelette or scrambled eggs. Or sardines with stewed tomatoes and chilli.

Dahl. Yes, cooked lentils. Delicious and simple, a batch of creamy dahl cooked with coconut milk and spices will last in the fridge all week. Eaten hot or cold, it takes as much time to serve as a bowl of cereal.

A breakfast frittata you prepared earlier… A frittata with eggs, plenty of vegetables and some cheese can be popped in the oven over the weekend then kept in the fridge. Zap a piece in the microwave for breakfast, or have it cold.

Fibre. Add fibre. Most people don't have even close to enough fibre. A tablespoon of psyllium husk in a large glass of water will give you a great start. Leafy green vegetables and pulses will make up your fibre quota during the day. There's more about psyllium and fibre generally in Chapter 4.

What about cereal?

Breakfast cereal is *too high in carbs, low in protein and absent of vegetables to be a good breakfast choice on its own.*

Most processed cereals, including many brands of muesli, are high in carbs with significant amounts of added sugar. Even the humble wheat biscuit made from wholegrain wheat is high in carbs, although at least these generally aren't coming from added sugar. Processed cereals usually include flavourings, preservatives and other additives.

Plain rolled oats and some brands of untoasted muesli have less than 60 g of carbs per 100 g, and sugars well under 10 g per 100 g, which makes them lower in carbs than other cereals. However, *none of the cereals is a good source of protein.*

If you're not ready to be separated from your cereal, then have a quarter of a cup of plain oats or lower-carb muesli and add a decent dollop of plain unsweetened yoghurt, nuts, and pumpkin or chia seeds, to build up the protein content.

> ### Morning exercise
>
> If you go to the gym, run, or do other aerobic exercise early in the morning, it's fine to have breakfast after you exercise. But notice what you're eating the day before! A recent study showed that people who plan to exercise first thing before breakfast, tend to eat more in the 24 hours beforehand.[13]

Some anti-breakfast excuses

I'm not hungry at breakfast time

It's important to eat at regular mealtimes. Breakfast is a regular meal from now on.

A few things will help with the 'no morning appetite':

- Stop eating at least four hours before bed and drink only water after that. If you still don't wake hungry, have your last meal earlier, and make it smaller.

- Start your new breakfast habit kindly – it can be very small and light, just make sure it's high in protein and fibre, with no refined carbs or sugar.

- Make a commitment. Make breakfast a promise to yourself.

I'm doing intermittent fasting

Intermittent fasting is an effective way to shed weight. But read the section on intermittent fasting later in this chapter to make sure you're getting the most out of it. It's not the same as skipping breakfast.

---

[13] Barutcu (2021) Planned morning aerobic exercise in a fasted state increases energy intake in the preceding 24 h.

If I eat breakfast, I'm starving just a couple of hours later

First – a breakfast that's high in refined carbs (e.g. toast and orange juice) is likely to leave you hungry, or wanting more carbs, soon after you've eaten. On the other hand, a high-protein, high-fibre breakfast with some fat will keep you satisfied for around three hours.

Second – being hungry three hours after breakfast is a sign that your metabolism is functioning as it should be, and hasn't 'shut down' because it thinks there's a famine on. Our insulin sensitivity and the amount of energy we burn after eating are both higher in the morning, indicating that our metabolism is optimised for eating in the earlier part of the day.

I don't have time…

You do have time. Breakfast doesn't need to be a full sit-down affair, and can be prepared while you're doing other things. If you don't have the prep time in the morning, get breakfast ready the night before. Then make five to 10 minutes for eating: just you and your body, connecting over breakfast. Making time for eating is a necessary act of self-love.

> ## Top tip – quick eggs
>
> In the evening, partly poach a couple of eggs – until they're still wobbly in the middle, but just set on the outside (about four minutes). Put them in a microwave safe container in the fridge. Next morning, zap them for 30 seconds, or slide them into a small pan of boiling water for a minute or so. Poached eggs, done.
>
> Or for the ultimate quick eggs, break two eggs into a cup, place a plate on top and microwave until they're done – just 40 seconds or so.

Find a breakfast you like, and stick to it

Breakfast is a solid start, every day, to your commitment to practise healthy eating habits. An excellent way to stick to a new habit is to automate it – take the guesswork and choice out of it. My advice is to have the same breakfast every day.

Have most of your food before 3 pm

Evidence shows that to reach and maintain a healthy weight, we should be eating most of our energy (calories), and especially most of our carbs, earlier in the day.

A large number of studies in recent years demonstrate that early eating leads to greater weight reduction and reduction in body fat, as well as significant improvements in markers of metabolic health, while later eating is associated with an increase in body fat and poorer metabolic health. There is also evidence that early eating increases our metabolism by generating significantly higher diet-induced thermogenesis than eating later in the day (more on metabolism in Chapter 7).

Make your evening meal early and light

There is strong evidence that eating later in the day, particularly in the evening, increases the likelihood of accumulating excess body fat. The larger and later our evening meals (or alcohol, sweetened drinks, milk and snacks), the more likely we are to gain fat.

Have a *light* evening meal, and finish it at least three to four hours before going to bed.

What is a 'light meal'?

It's small. Clench your fist. That's the maximum size of a light meal – minus salad or non-starchy vegetables. Add up to another fist-size of salad or non-starchy vegetables. No dressing, apart from a drizzle of oil and vinegar that you mixed yourself.

It's mostly protein and some fat, and either no carbs, or a very small amount of high-quality carbs.

Light meal ideas

- Stir-fry vegetables, with a protein source. Whether you're vegetarian or not, adding pulses (e.g. chickpeas or soybeans) provides high-quality carbs with extra protein and fibre too.

- Tuna with green beans, broccoli, peas and red capsicum.

- Boiled eggs and green salad with raw almonds.

- Whatever your family's having, without the carbs.

  » If it's tuna mornay, remove your serve before adding pasta and white sauce.

  » If it's spaghetti bolognaise, have bolognaise and salad, without the pasta.

  » If it's sausages with mashed potatoes and salad, eliminate the mash.

  » If it's stir-fry, take out your share before adding noodles, and say no to rice.

For even better results, further reduce the size of your last meal, and a few times a week, finish eating by 4 pm. This is the ***Five for Life Fast*** – it's outlined later in the chapter.

Then stop. No night-time snacking

We burn more fat when we *fast overnight*. So choose that your sleep time will be spent fat burning, not fat storing. After your last meal – no evening or night-time snacks, including alcohol or other calorie-containing drinks.

But what if I'm hungry?

Many of us feel like reaching for a sweet or savoury snack an hour or so after dinner. It's an eating habit rather than true hunger, and you're going to make a new habit: no eating after the evening meal. It will get easier over time.

One reason we seek food in the evening is that our biological clocks are stuck in ancient times, telling us to get ready for a fast… because who knows when we'll eat again? This habit worked to help keep cave-men safe from starvation, but now we know exactly when we'll eat again – the very next day. If you have been on diets in the past, your unconscious brain will be particularly concerned about the possibility of another famine, and will try prompting you to eat in the evening to store more fat.

Think of an after-dinner urge to eat as an ideal opportunity to 'just say no'; to support your body to burn more fat, using your natural night-time fast to help.

Eating early vs. family life and other realities

Chances are that this new habit – eating early to support your circadian rhythm – won't come easily. Our lifestyles and eating habits have largely evolved to match a 9-to-5 work routine. Our main meal has had to fit around work, school or other activities, which means we do it at the end of the day. Even when we aren't working, we tend to stick to this meal timing through habit, and because it's the way most people in Australia still eat, which means it's more sociable. And being social is an important part of our eating habits.

Sitting down to share a meal with those we love is a precious part of life and we should do it whenever we can. If we're fortunate enough to come home to a meal that's been prepared for us, and to eat it with those who care for us, that's cause for quiet joy.

But there's no need to have large quantities. Take a small serve, eat it slowly and make it last. Explain why you're eating this way, and especially if you have younger children, be confident that this is modelling healthy eating habits for an older person. Let children understand that as we get older and stop growing, it's healthier to have most of our food earlier in the day.

And remember that blessed are the leftovers. Breakfast or lunch the next day.

Shift working and night owls

Being up and about and eating when nature would prefer us to be sleeping directly disrupts our circadian rhythm and carries a heavy health burden – literally. It makes us fat, and is associated with significantly increased risk of heart disease and other serious illnesses. Chapter 8 looks into managing weight if you're a shift worker or night owl.

Does it have to be like this forever?

To reduce weight, stick to the four steps of the 'circadian sync' *90% of the time*. To maintain weight, stick to this eating method *most of the time*.

- *Eat breakfast* every day for the rest of your life (barring something extraordinary, of course).

- *Eat most of your calories before 3 pm.*

- *Stick to an early, small dinner as often as possible*. Remember that the later you're eating, the smaller the meal needs to be. Keep a close watch, and if you notice your weight or waist measurement creeping up, revert to *earlier, smaller evening meals*.

- *No late-night snacking*. It's an unhealthy habit – kick it forever. Once you reach your target weight, make the odd exception (ideally no more than once per month) if you're out with friends or on a special occasion.

The *Five for Life Fast* described at the end of this chapter is a variation on the circadian sync, combining what we know about the benefits of both intermittent fasting and breakfast.

> **HABIT HELPERS – EAT EARLY**
>
> *Eat early.* Eat breakfast, eat most before 3 pm, and *make the last meal the least, with nothing later*. Of all the tips in this book, *this is the most effective*. If you do nothing else (apart

from drastically reducing sugar!), do this. Check out the *Five for Life Fast* in the next section, which extends the 'eat early' habit.

Talk to yourself. Write it down and say it out loud: 'I have a tiny amount at dinner'; 'I don't eat after dinner'; 'I've stopped eating for the day. I choose to burn fat now, not store more.'

Ritualise end-of-eating. Develop some 'end-of-eating-day' signals:

- clean your teeth
- have a pot of herbal tea, unsweetened and free of caffeine and other stimulants.

Take up an empty-belly activity for the time you usually head to the kitchen for nibbles. Try yoga, swimming or singing.

If ***night-time snacking*** is a challenge for you, Chapter 10 has more ideas on how to change.

REFLECTIONS

Sync your circadian rhythm

- Do you normally eat breakfast? If not, why not? What will you do to start a life-time breakfast habit?

- How will you make sure to eat most of your daily food before 3 pm?

- What time do you normally have your last meal? What changes will you make to your routine to finish eating earlier in the day?

- Do you tend to snack, or drink alcohol, milk, or juice after your last meal? What will you do to end night-time snacking?

Intermittent fasting

Intermittent fasting has been the subject of increasing research in recent years, and much has been said and written on the topic both scientifically and in the popular press.

Done properly, it's a good thing

Many studies now show that intermittent fasting, done properly, usually helps people shed excess weight and body fat, including visceral fat. It's also likely to improve our health in other important ways, reducing blood pressure, fasting glucose and cholesterol levels, and reducing systemic inflammation.

There are many forms of intermittent fasting, with periods of complete fasting or reduced energy intake followed by periods of unrestricted intake. The '5:2' method is a well-known example: five days of the week you eat normally, and on each of the two fasting days (which can be consecutive or not), you eat only 25–30% of your usual energy intake.

For women?

Limited studies have been done on different types of fasting specifically in women, but what exists indicates that for hormonal reasons, longer fasts may not be suitable for most women, and time-restricted eating with plenty of daily protein is the better option. Intermittent fasting also isn't recommended for people with a history of eating disorders.

Time-restricted eating

Time-restricted eating is a newly popular way to do intermittent fasting, with studies showing it can be effective for reducing body fat. It's certainly the easiest and, therefore, probably the most sustainable. It's also a good option for most women.

Time-restricted eating means limiting the period during which you eat *each day*, so that the 'eating window' is anywhere from just four hours, up to 12 hours per day. For example, people refer to the '16:8' or '14:10' diets, where the larger number is the fasting period, and the smaller number is the eating window. If you have breakfast at 8 am and finish eating by 6 pm that evening, you're doing a '14:10' intermittent fast, fasting for the 14 hours from 6 pm until 8 am the next day. For most people, the shorter the eating window, the more effective the fast appears to be.

One important thing that is evident from recent studies, and discussed in the previous section, is that eating in sync with our circadian rhythm is essential for maintaining a healthy weight long term. And this basically means 'eating early'. So if you want to reap all the benefits of time-restricted eating, *the time during which you fast should match your circadian rhythm*. Aim for a 14-hour fast that ends at breakfast.

The ***Five for Life Fast*** described at the end of this section combines time-restricted eating, eating early, and real life, into a doable and effective eating plan.

Breakfast skipping

Breakfast skipping is a popular way to increase an overnight fast. Lots of people do it, and have shed weight eating this way, at least in the short term. It's an attractive option because it's compatible with family and social life (you can still have an evening meal and drinks). But as we saw in the previous section, the evidence and odds are stacked against it being a safe and effective long-term strategy for reaching and maintaining a healthy weight.

The bulk of the large population-based studies show that for most people, skipping breakfast doesn't help shed fat, and if you make it a habit, you're more likely to gain fat.

In addition to the epidemiological studies, controlled clinical trials of time-restricted eating and the effects of skipping breakfast show there are distinct metabolic advantages from eating breakfast. Well-designed controlled trials since about 2014 demonstrate that those who eat breakfast and fast from early evening *burn more fat and have better fasting glucose levels and insulin sensitivity*, than those who skip breakfast and eat between 12 noon and 8 pm.

Fasting vs. 'crash diets'

Fasting, even extreme fasting, can be a healthy way to shed fat while maintaining lean muscle if done properly and not for too long (preferably under professional supervision, if you want to try it). But it's important not to confuse fasting with crash diets, which also advocate very low food intake. The difference between fasting and a crash diet is in *what* you eat.

A daily diet of 800 calories worth of cabbage soup or fruit juice will leave you seriously deficient in nutrients. On the other hand, 800 calories of high-quality protein, vegetables and fats will leave you perfectly healthy. Possibly hungry (800 calories is very low), but nevertheless your organs and body systems will still be functioning properly.

A crash diet is any eating plan that involves cutting out a food group (sugar is not a 'food group'!). So 'no carbs', 'no fat', or 'fruit only' is a crash diet. A crash diet is also one that restricts energy to less than about 1,200 calories per day for more than a short fasting period.

Our body needs particular nutrients to function properly. We need a range of foods, and enough protein, fat and good-quality carbs (including fibre), to get all those nutrients. So please – don't crash diet. Your body doesn't deserve to be treated that way.

> ### Ketogenesis – not crashing
>
> A ketogenic diet is very high in fat with moderate to high protein, and less than 50 g of carbs per day, mostly from non-starchy vegetables. The radical reduction in carbs activates different metabolic pathways (ketosis), so the body accesses its energy needs from dietary fat and stored body fat.

There is strong evidence that a ketogenic diet is a safe and effective antidote to overweight and obesity, and for treating and potentially reversing type 2 diabetes and metabolic syndrome. If you're interested in a keto diet, speak to a dietitian who can help you do it safely and effectively. A keto diet isn't safe for a small number of people with specific health conditions.

The main drawback with a ketogenic diet is that it's difficult to maintain long term.[14] Most people don't keep it up forever and rebound to pre-diet eating habits, putting all the weight back on, plus more. The key is to have built up healthy eating habits before, during and after a keto diet, to support you when you return to a higher (but not too high) level of carbs.

If you don't think a full keto diet is for you, a diet that's simply low in carbs (less than about 130 g per day, with little or no refined carbs) also has proven health benefits. Chapter 4 outlines this style of eating.

Long-term calorie restriction

Low-calorie diets reduce our resting metabolic rate, which conserves energy and reduces the production of the free radicals that damage our cells. If the diet itself contains all required nutrients, evidence indicates that a long-term, very low-calorie diet may reduce weight, increase lifespan by up to five years, and improve overall health during your longer life.

There's a catch of course – the caloric restriction needed to achieve these results is around 15–30% less energy than your body is normally considered to need, as a permanent measure. It's definitely not for everyone! Most people would find it difficult to live in this way, not least because it leaves little room for the social

---

[14] There's also some debate about whether it's good for your kidneys, liver and bones over the long term. There are competing studies and no consensus at this point.

aspects of food and eating. The other catch is that the reduced metabolic rate (even if you do this for a short stint) *is a long-term effect*. This means that if you revert to higher calorie intake, your body will be very keen to store the additional energy as body fat.

If you're interested in this fairly radical approach to a longer life, it's important to consult a dietitian before you embark on it.

The Five for Life Fast (aka the fasting circadian sync)

The *Five for Life Fast* is an easy yet effective way to do time-restricted eating to reach your happy weight, or use a modified version of it to maintain your weight. This method makes the most of the evidence on eating breakfast, intermittent fasting and eating in sync with your circadian rhythm, while acknowledging that finishing eating by 4 pm *every* day isn't feasible for many of us.

How to do it

1. ***Fuel-up before four***. Have breakfast and lunch every day. These need to be proper meals. Chapter 4 has more about building good meals, but the short story is that breakfast and lunch should each include at least 20–30 g protein, lots of non-starchy vegetables, and plenty of healthy fats. Have at least 80% of your daily energy intake before 4 pm.

2. ***End before eight***. Eat a light meal in the early evening, four days of the week. Make it as early as you can – close to 6 pm and no later than 8 pm.

3. ***Leave three free***. Three times each week, don't have an evening meal. Have your last energy intake by 4 pm, making sure that you've clocked up all or most of your daily non-starchy vegetable and minimum protein requirements. Then no snacking, or drinks other than water, after that. Busy weeknights that keep your mind off food are ideal evenings to 'leave free'.

And that's all.

If you find yourself accidentally eating late one night, don't panic. A common response to feeling that we've 'fallen off the wagon' is to skip breakfast the next day to somehow make up for eating late the night before, but it doesn't work like that. The best thing is to continue to be kind to yourself, and plan things differently for the next day.

The following morning, get up and look at yourself in the mirror. You're still you! Beautiful and worthy. Then go and have a few glasses of water and a small, high-protein breakfast, because regular meals, especially breakfast, are essential to long-term healthy weight maintenance.

Recap – When to eat

What's the problem? We eat when we aren't hungry. We eat too much. And we eat too late in the day.

Feel it. Recognise your own hunger signals. Ask '*Am I hungry?*' before eating.

Stay regular. Establish a regular eating routine and stick to it as much as possible.

Keep it small. Reduce portion sizes to recalibrate your brain's understanding of when it has had enough. Use smaller plates and smaller cutlery.

Some for now, some for later. If you're used to serving a larger portion at dinner, practise dividing it into thirds. Two thirds now, one third for a light meal or snack another time.

Out of sight. Serve up, then pack leftovers away in the fridge and pantry.

Signal it. Clean your teeth after eating a meal or snack, to signal that you've had enough for now.

Do the Fasting Circadian Sync. Follow the *Five for Life Fast* for an easy and effective way to practise time-restricted eating.

CHAPTER FOUR

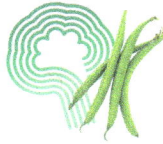

WHAT TO EAT

One of the most overwhelming things for a lot of people is figuring out what to eat, and especially what *not* to eat. If you're anything like me, you grew up thinking that cereal and a glass of orange juice was a healthy breakfast.

So just a warning – this is a long chapter, because there's a lot to say about *what to eat, and what to avoid*.

You don't have to look far to see many different opinions about the best things to eat if you want to become healthier, lighter, and stay that way. Well-known diet options include keto, paleo, vegetarian, vegan, veg-and-fish (pescatarian), meat-and-dairy, and Mediterranean.

I'm not going to go into detailed pros and cons of different diets, as there's no need to get so complicated. I'll just keep it simple, because it really is. But here's the secret: no one, least of all advertisers, makes money out of that idea. And that's a big part of the 'what to eat' problem.

The Five for Life approach can be applied to any diet provided it *emphasises vegetables (especially greens), includes sufficient protein and 'good' fat, and limits sugar and other refined carbs*.

In this chapter, we'll cover:

- some *food basics* – the short story on eating the right food, what food is 'made of' (the macronutrients), and what happens when we eat

- the importance of *vegetables, protein, fat and carbs* – they each have a section of their own

- the *'danger zone'* – food that's guaranteed to prevent us from reaching and keeping our happy weight.

Need-to-know: the food basics

What to eat? The short story

Eat food that functions! Real food fuels our body with what it needs. The right food is dense in nutrients – vitamins and minerals, protein, 'good' fat and fibre.

To reduce weight safely and permanently, focus on these four principles:

1. Eat a lot more greens and other non-starchy vegetables. Whatever you like! Salad leaves, broccoli, zucchini, cauliflower, capsicum, tomatoes, green beans and the rest. These foods are high in fibre, vitamins, minerals and trace elements. Add fermented vegetables like sauerkraut and kimchi, too.

2. Eat plenty of protein and fat (unprocessed). It's essential for good health to get enough protein every day. Meat, poultry, fish and eggs are concentrated sources of protein, as are pulses such as chickpeas, dried beans, lentils and soy. It's also important to have enough fat from healthy, unprocessed sources. Get *most* of your fat from vegetables (e.g. raw nuts and seeds, avocado, olives), cold-pressed olive oil and other cold-pressed oils, and fish. It's fine to have some fats from animal sources too, such as eggs, meat, butter and cheese.

3. Reduce carbs. Unprocessed carbs like starchy vegetables (e.g. potatoes, sweet potato, sweet corn and pumpkin), fruit and whole grains (e.g. rolled oats, quinoa and wild rice) are good for us in *smaller amounts*, but they offer little that we don't get from non-starchy vegetables, or from fat and protein sources. What they do add are extra calories in the form of sugars and starch. We do need carbs in our diet, but not much.

4. Cut right down, or cut out, processed carbs, sugar, fillers and fake food. This includes 'danger zone' food, designed to keep us *wanting more* even if we aren't hungry. I'm not just talking about highly processed foods and added sugar, but also carbs made from refined flours – cakes, biscuits, pastries, and most breads, pasta and breakfast cereal.

To help work out what to eat, and how much, I use a traffic light system, which I hope will make it simpler to remember. It's on page 98.

The takeaway on takeaway...

Sellers of ready-made food rely on it being both tasty and convenient. *Not* healthy. Ready-made food and food ready in a hurry (fast food) is almost invariably based on poor-quality carbs such as bread, potato, rice or pasta, along with added sugar, salt and processed oils.

There's no way around it – this stuff will make you accumulate fat.

Protein, fat, carbs... what are they exactly?

Everything we eat is made of protein, fat or carbs: the three macronutrients. They provide the main building blocks our body needs to function, and we get all of our energy (measured in units of calories or kilojoules[15]) from them.

---

15   In this book I use calories. There are about 4.2 kJ to a calorie, if you want to convert.

Alcohol is also classed as a macronutrient because it provides energy. We don't need alcohol to function, so it's not included in this chapter. It's an important topic when it comes to our weight, though, so alcohol has a section of its own in Chapter 5.

Most foods are a combination of at least some carbs, proteins and fats, but are dominant in one or two of those. And some foods are almost entirely one form of macronutrient. For example:

- *Sugar* is pure carbs – no protein or fat.

- *Fruit* is more than 80–90% carbs, with small amounts of protein and virtually no fat.

- *Plant oils and animal fats* (e.g. olive oil and butter) are almost pure fat, with nil or negligible protein and no carbs.

- *Meat and fish* are almost entirely protein, with no carbs and some fat. Fat levels vary widely depending on the type of animal and cut.

- *Nuts and seeds* are mostly fat, but also contain significant protein.

- *Pulses* are mostly carbs, but also contain significant protein.

- *Milk* is nearly half carbs, the remainder an even balance of protein and fat.[16] *Yoghur*t is lower in carbs and higher in fat and protein than milk. (Non-dairy substitutes have very different profiles – less protein and more carbs than the dairy equivalent.)

In this book, food is referred to as:

- *Protein* if at least 15% of its energy value comes from protein. *E.g. lean meat and poultry, fish and other seafood, eggs, cottage cheese, pulses (such as chickpeas and lentils), tofu and tempeh, nuts and seeds.*

- *Carbs* if at least 50% of its energy value comes from carbs. *E.g. all fruit, all starchy vegetables (potato, sweet potato, sweet corn), all pulses (chickpeas, lentils and kidney beans), all grains and*

---

[16] It's a myth that a cup of low-fat milk has more carbs than a cup of full-cream milk (check the food labels to compare carbs per 100 ml). The weight of the fat missing from the skim version is made up with water, or sometimes with more protein in the form of non-fat milk solids.

flour (wheat, oats, barley, rice), all forms of sugar, and all products made mostly from grains or sugar, such as bread, pasta, cake and confectionery.

- **Fat** if at least 70% of its energy value comes from fat.
  E.g. nuts and seeds, all oils, animal fat, vegetable fat, olives, avocado, butter, cream and cheese.

Where does fibre fit?

Fibre is a form of carbs. However, as fibre is mostly not digested, it provides virtually no energy. Generally when we talk about carbs, we don't mean fibre.

Even though it doesn't supply energy, fibre is an essential part of our diet and it helps to reduce weight and keep it off. We take a closer look at the importance of fibre later in this chapter.

What about vitamins and minerals?

Apart from protein, fat and carbs, food also contains vitamins, minerals and trace elements. As we need these substances in very small amounts, they're known as micronutrients – see Chapter 7 for more on this.

What happens when we eat?

Breaking it all down

When we eat or drink, our body breaks down the macronutrients in our food. The protein components are converted to amino acids, the fats to fatty acids, and the carbs to glucose. Glucose, amino acids and fatty acids play multiple and complementary roles in our bodies.

- **Amino acids** are our building blocks, used to make muscle tissue and to make other proteins that our body needs, including hormones.
- **Fatty acids** are used to make cell walls and hormones, as well as for other purposes.

- *Glucose* is used (very rapidly) to provide our cells with fuel. Great if you're about to go for a run. Not necessarily great otherwise.

Too much glucose in our bloodstream is dangerous, so as soon as levels rise – which happens shortly after eating carbs – our body needs to quickly either use up the glucose as energy, or deal with it another way. The 'other way' is by storing it – a little is stored in our liver and muscles as glycogen, but mostly it's converted then stored as fat, in our fat cells.

The carb effect

We convert different types of carbs into blood glucose at different rates. Foods high in refined sugar and starch, and low in fibre (including sugary food, flour, most bread, white rice and potatoes) are converted quickly. *Unprocessed carbs* that are high in fibre (e.g. non-starchy vegetables, pulses and unprocessed whole grains) are converted more slowly.

The faster a carb is converted to glucose, the higher its 'glycaemic index' (GI).[17] The higher the GI of our carbs, or the more carbs we eat in a meal overall, the more our blood sugar will rise, leading to greater fat storage.

The final destination for any unused fuel – whether its original source was carbs, protein or fat – is storage as body fat. However, we are more likely to store the excess fuel from carbs as body fat, because the primary job of carbs is to produce glucose – which is 100% energy.

Carbs, especially sugar and refined carbs, are the main cause of fat we store if we eat too much.

Reducing weight is about using more, storing less

Without going into the (very) complex chemistry of metabolism, to reduce body fat we need to do two things:

---

[17] The section in this chapter on carbs, and Appendix B, have more detail on the GI.

- *Use up more stored body fat* as energy by reducing carb intake, maintaining the right daily protein intake, and fasting overnight (from as early as you can).

- *Reduce new body fat* stored each day by keeping blood sugar low and stable. This means avoiding high-GI carbs (e.g. sugar, white bread and other refined flour products, potatoes and rice), and not overeating.

Food processing

The protein, fat or carb content of our food is only part of the 'eat the right food' puzzle, and it may not be the most important part. We also need to know *how much the food has been processed*.

Processed food has been altered in some way from its natural form: maybe cooked, ground up, split into different parts or mixed with other substances. Some foods are barely processed (e.g. eggs, fruit, vegetables, nuts and seeds), while some have minimal processing. Butter, plain dairy yoghurt and canned beans, for instance, have had basic processing, but they're perfectly healthy.

Highly processed carbs and fats are often referred to as 'refined'. For example, refined flour is made from grains whose outer skin and inner germ have been removed, leaving just the white, starchy part. Refined oil is created from highly processed seed or bean oil.

Then there's *ultra-processed food*. This is the stuff you couldn't make at home. It includes highly refined and synthetic ingredients such as artificial flavourings and colourings, texture enhancers, modified starch, protein isolate, hydrogenated oils, stabilisers and emulsifiers. It may also have been extruded or moulded into shapes.

Ultra-processed food isn't necessarily easy to recognise without reading the ingredients, but there's a lot of it around. It's often colourful, relatively inexpensive and over-packaged, but not always. Items such as baby foods, pre-prepared meals and products targeted at dieters such as meal substitutes and protein bars are also typically ultra-processed.

Highly processed and ultra-processed food is dangerous, and there is growing evidence that it's making us fatter and sicker.

In a recent Australian study, two groups were offered food of the same calories, and with the same ratio of protein, carbs and fat, and allowed to eat as much as they liked. For the first fortnight, one group's food was more than 80% highly processed, while the other group had no highly processed food. In the second fortnight, the groups swapped so that each group completed both types of diet. While eating the highly processed food, participants ate significantly more, ate more quickly, and put on an average of nearly a kilo (400 g of which was body fat) in the space of two weeks. But they all *shed* nearly a kilo (including 300 g of body fat) when eating the unprocessed food.[18] Apart from this marked effect on weight, studies also show that ultra-processed food is associated with heart disease, metabolic syndrome and diabetes, as well as cancer and depression.

Traffic lights – the good, the bad and the ordinary

To make it simpler to choose the right food, Five for Life uses a traffic light system:

- *Green zone.* Eat mostly from this zone. Foods in this zone are unprocessed or have minimal processing and no added sugar.

- *Amber zone.* Foods in this zone are fine to eat, in smaller quantities than green zone foods. Food in this zone is mostly unprocessed, or has had minimal processing.

  The amber zone also includes low-processed proteins, as some of these aren't too bad. For example, good-quality sausages are simply ground meat, plus a small amount of bulker such as rice flour, and herbs and spices packed in natural casing. Check the ingredients. The more there are (especially things you don't recognise), the more the food slips into the red zone. As a

---

[18] Hall (2019) Ultra-processed diets cause excess calorie intake and weight gain: an inpatient randomized controlled trial of ad libitum food intake.

general rule, enjoy good-quality, low-processed protein in small quantities, and infrequently.

- **Red zone**. Eat as little from this zone as possible. *The less red zone food you have, the easier it will be to reach and stay at your ideal weight.* This zone includes all sweetened and highly processed, refined foods.

- **Danger zone**. Foods in this zone are associated with symptoms of addiction, and are a serious risk to your weight and general health. They're mostly starchy carbs prepared with poor-quality fat and added sugar or salt (or both).

The Traffic Light Table is on the next page.

How much do we need?

We need some carbs, some protein, and some fat, every day. But *how much* we have of each makes a difference to how easy it is to reduce weight, and stay at a happy weight.

There are different opinions and government guidelines about the 'right' balance to shed excess weight and maintain a healthy weight. Some of these are out of date in terms of carb and fat needs, and don't reflect current research on the role of carbs in weight gain.

To shed excess fat and keep it off, there's no need to be preoccupied with precise macronutrient ratios. Eating mostly from the green zone, just focus first on getting plenty of protein, then a lot of non-starchy vegetables and enough high-quality fat. Finally, choose some amber zone carbs. Be cautious about eating from the red or danger zones.

THE TRAFFIC LIGHT TABLE – WHAT TO EAT

	PROTEIN	FAT	CARBS
GREEN ZONE (eat most)	**Animal sources (unprocessed)** e.g. lean meat and poultry, fish and other seafood, eggs, cottage cheese **Plant sources (unprocessed)** e.g. pulses (peas, chickpeas, lentils, beans), plain tofu and tempeh, nuts and seeds	**Fats from plants and fish (unprocessed)** e.g. olive oil, avocado, raw nuts and seeds, naturally oily fish such as salmon and mackerel	**Non-starchy vegetables** e.g. all salad vegetables, broccoli, cabbage, zucchini, cauliflower, dark leafy greens **Pulses** e.g. chickpeas, lentils, kidney beans, black beans, butter beans, yellow split peas
AMBER ZONE (limit quantities)	**Low-processed meats** e.g. high-quality sausages or burger patties (minimal filler and no artificial flavouring), ham and bacon with minimal additives **Low-processed plant-based protein** e.g. low-additive soy or seitan products or meat-free patties	**Fats from animals, coconut and palm (unprocessed)** e.g. butter, cream, cheese, lard, coconut oil and palm oil	**Starchy vegetables** e.g. potatoes, parsnip, sweet corn **Fruit** all fruit (up to 2 serves/day) **Whole grains and wholegrain products** e.g. quinoa, oats, barley, wild rice and brown rice, pasta or bread made with wholegrain flour **Dairy** unsweetened milk and yoghurt

| RED ZONE (avoid) | Highly processed meat or meat-free products
e.g. low-quality sausages and processed meat products including processed ham and meat substitutes

Protein processed with red zone carbs or fats
e.g. pies, nuggets, battered and crumbed items | Processed fats, trans fats and fats from the deep-fryer
check the label on packaged food, and avoid deep-fried food and refined vegetable oils | Sugar
e.g. table sugar, cane sugar, concentrated fruit sugar, syrup (such as maple and agave) and fruit juices

Refined grains and refined-grain products (including gluten-free)
e.g. white rice, bread, pasta, cakes, biscuits, most breakfast cereals

Dairy
sweetened milk or yoghurt |
| DANGER ZONE | A hyper-flavoursome combination of starchy carbs, fat, and added sugar and/or salt
e.g. potato chips and crisps, pizza, cakes, biscuits, pastries, donuts and most desserts

Many red zone foods fall into the danger zone too. | | |

Download a printable PDF of The Traffic Light table from the Five for Life website.

To put a bit more detail around 'how much':

- *Plenty of protein.* At least 1 g (and up to 2 g) of protein per kilo of your own body weight each day. For example if you weigh 60 kg, you'll need at least 60 g and up to 120 g protein each day. A piece of chicken or meat the size of your palm contains about 30 g protein, depending on the size of your palm. A cup of cooked lentils contains about 10 g.

- *A lot of non-starchy vegetables.* At least 400 g of vegetables every day (not counting potatoes, sweet potatoes, pumpkin, parsnip, sweet corn or pulses).

- *Sufficient 'good' fat.* Between 50 and 100 g of fat per day, depending on your total energy needs. This should come mostly from olive oil and other cold-pressed oils, avocado, raw nuts and seeds, and oily fish. Fat from other animal sources is fine in smaller quantities.

- *Finally, look at carbs.* Ideally, your protein sources will include some pulses, and these are also an excellent source of high-quality carbs. If you're vegetarian or vegan, pulses and higher protein whole grains will be two of your main protein sources, so you may not need any more carbs. To reduce weight, aim for a maximum of 150 g of carbs per day for smaller-framed people (including most women), or 200 g per day for men or those with a larger frame. Choose high-quality carbs that are nutrient rich and high in fibre: pulses, or small quantities of whole grains, whole fruit, or starchy vegetables.

- *Drastically limit sugars and refined grains and flours.* We don't need any of these. They make us fat, and they make us crave more sugar. The main reason so many of us are overweight is because this form of low-quality carb is all around. It's cheap to produce, and it's addictive. Food manufacturers love it.

That's really all you need to know.

Macro-counting

'Macro-counting' is the practice of choosing a ratio of protein, fat and carbs for your total daily energy intake, then tracking your intake against that ratio. Some people find it helps them maintain a good balance of macronutrients – enough protein and fats, and not too many carbs.

If you want to use this method, be willing to weigh food and use a calculator a lot, but most importantly *mind the quality of your nutrients* – they're not all the same! In particular, *carb quality matters*. Choose mostly from the green zone, with smaller quantities from the amber zone. Avoid the red and danger zones.

The rest of this chapter details *how* to get more vegetables, plenty of protein, sufficient good fat, and the right amount of (the right) carbs.

Last, we look at the 'wrong carbs' – *sugary and danger zone food* – the most common cause of overweight and obesity.

HABIT HELPERS – EAT FOOD WITH FUNCTION

Know what you're eating. Recognise the sources of protein, fat and carbs in the food you eat. Find out where the added sugar, refined flour and grains are lurking in your everyday diet.

Front of mind. Print out the Traffic Light Table from the Five for Life website and keep it somewhere you'll see it all the time – on the fridge or kitchen bench.

Think it. Meal planning and prep will take a little longer if you've been used to including processed food or takeaway. But dedicating precious time to your loyal body is a gift, not a nuisance. And meal prep gets quicker and easier with practice. (Chapter 11 has more on this.)

Say it. '*Sugar makes me ill*'.

Do it. Eat more vegetables, plenty of protein, sufficient fat, and a small amount of whole grains, fruit and starchy vegetables. Cut out as much sugar and refined flour as possible. And avoid takeaway food until you reach your target weight.

> ## REFLECTIONS
>
> ### *Meals and snacks*
>
> - What do you enjoy eating? What are your favourite non-starchy vegetables, favourite sources of protein, and sources of 'good' fat?
> - What is a typical breakfast, lunch and dinner for you?
> - Do you tend to snack? How often, and what do you have? Do you recognise your snacking triggers?
> - What small changes will you make to shift more of your eating to the green zone?
>
> ### *Keep a food diary for a week*
>
> - List everything you eat, and approximately how much.
> - Think about why you made each choice. When did you eat, and where?
> - Notice how much protein, vegetables, fibre and water you had each day. Notice the type and quantity of carbs, using the Traffic Light Table to categorise them. Notice how much of what you ate was processed, or highly processed.
> - Repeat the process every month or so, and compare to see what's changed over time.

More vegetables

The short story on vegetables

Eating more vegetables, especially greens, is essential to reaching and staying at your ideal weight.

Vegetables are our most important source of *fibre, vitamins and minerals, and high-quality carbs*. For vegetarians and vegans, they're also the most important source of protein. They also help fill us up, without excess calories.

Eat as many non-starchy vegetables as you can. They should make up the bulk of every meal. Think green beans, broccoli, spinach, kale, bok choy, tomatoes, cucumber, capsicum and salad greens.

Limit your starchy vegetables: potatoes, sweet potatoes, sweet corn and pumpkin.

Avoid dressing or sauce on your vegetables unless it's home-made, with no sweeteners.

Eat more fibre. Use natural psyllium husk as a calorie-free fibre supplement.

Non-starchy vegetables: eat most

Greens – not called superfood for nothing

Greens are so densely packed with the good stuff, and with exceptionally low carb content, they need to be our priority. Include plenty of anything green in your daily meals:

- kale, spinach, silverbeet and chard
- Asian greens, bok choy, choy sum and tatsoi
- salad greens, bitter greens, brussels sprouts and bean sprouts
- zucchini, broccoli, asparagus and cabbage.

Include those other greens too – seaweed! Find it in Asian groceries, and increasingly in other supermarkets too. In all its varieties, it's delicious in soups and salads, as a garnish, or as a snack (e.g. kelp jerky or thin, crispy nori).

Also eat your reds, whites, oranges, pinks...

Eating a range of colourful vegetables ensures we get almost all our vitamin and mineral needs. Aim for a plate of colour, as the plant world has amazing variety. Cauliflower, tomatoes, carrots, eggplant, pumpkin, capsicum, radishes, swedes… The different colours are partly due to the different types of polyphenols – compounds in vegetables and fruit that are extraordinarily good for us.

> ### Digestive upset? Brassicas and bum burps
>
> Many vegetables in the brassica family (e.g. cabbage, cauliflower and broccoli) contain a fair bit of fructans, a type of fermenting carb that can upset some people's digestive systems.
>
> If you think this might be you, check out some of the online information about FODMAPs foods (an acronym for Fermentable Oligosaccharides, Disaccharides, Mono-saccharides And Polyols) and see which type of brassicas might be okay in smaller servings. You'll probably be able to build up tolerance over time, so they're not gone forever.

How much? A lot

The World Health Organization recommends we have at least 400 g of non-starchy vegetables every day. It's a lot, and it means eating vegetables at every meal, and with snacks too.

> ### Worth their weight...
>
> - 1 medium head of broccoli (stalk trimmed) = 400 g
> - 1 cup of mixed salad vegetables (e.g. cucumber, tomato, radish and capsicum) = 130 g
> - 1 cup of salad leaves, loosely packed (e.g. lettuce, radicchio, baby spinach or rocket) = 30 g

Cook some things first – kale and other dark, leafy greens

Kale is an absolute powerhouse in terms of its nutritional value. Eating kale every day significantly boosts our intake of vitamins

A, C, B6 and K, calcium, iron, magnesium and antioxidants. It's high in fibre and very low in carbs. It's tasty and extremely versatile – use it in salads, fry it on its own with salt and pepper or other vegetables, add it to frittata, soup, stir-fry, lasagne or stew; make it into roasted chips or puree it to add to pesto.

Although it is delicious raw, you should *mostly eat kale lightly cooked*.

Kale and other dark, leafy greens, including spinach, silverbeet and chard, contains oxalic acid. Oxalic acid prevents us properly absorbing some minerals including calcium, magnesium and iron. Easily reduce oxalic acid by briefly steaming, or even just wilting, the leaves in hot water. Or add them to the rest of the meal just before the end of cooking.

High-carb vegetables: limit quantity

Some vegetables are high in carbs because they're high in sugar or starch, or both. This doesn't mean they're 'bad' for you, but do eat less of these than your non-starchy vegetables. ***Count high-carb and starchy vegetables as if they were grains, rather than greens.***

Eat up to one fistful of high-carb vegetables per day. There are two categories of high-carb vegetables – high starch and high sugar.

Starchy vegetables

The high starch vegetables are:

- potato and sweet potato
- sweet corn
- parsnips
- pumpkin
- garden peas.

Their starch content is in that order – potatoes and sweet corn have the most, peas least.

Sweet vegetables

The sweet vegetables (more than 5% sugar by weight) are beetroot and onions. Carrots are also a sweeter vegetable, with about half the sugar content of beetroot and onions.

In terms of how much to eat, treat sweet vegetables somewhere in between starchy and non-starchy vegetables.

Pulses

Pulses (e.g. kidney beans, chickpeas and lentils) are a special type of vegetable. Although they're high in starch, more than 30% of this is resistant starch, which is mostly not digested and acts as a nutrient for our gut biota. Pulses are also high in fibre and protein, slowing down the carb hit and reducing the chance of excess energy being stored as body fat, and counting towards daily protein intake. They're also high in valuable B vitamins, magnesium, zinc, iron and potassium.

Aim for around ½ cup a day (or a cup in a meal three or four times per week). If you're vegetarian, have at least a cup per day. A good way to have more pulses is to substitute: *decrease bread, rice, pasta and potatoes, and replace with pulses*.

If pulses give you gut issues, soak and rinse them well before using. Increase the amount you have slowly, starting with just a serve a week.

Soybean in your salad for something different

One cup of edamame beans (fresh young soybeans) provides 18 g of protein, your entire folate (vitamin B9) needs, and about half your daily vitamin K, as well as 8 g of fibre and a significant dose of magnesium and phosphorus.

And they're delicious on their own sprinkled with some salt and pepper, or added to salads.

Packing more veggies into your day

Don't just save veggies for dinner; it's a common habit and should definitely be ditched. You just can't get enough vegetables in the day unless you eat them at other meals and for snacks too.

For breakfast

Have a vegetable and protein-based breakfast. Some of my favourites are:

- poached or boiled eggs with wilted kale or spinach
- sardines or mackerel on a bed of steamed or fried mixed vegetables
- a veg-filled omelette.

If you've been in a 'breakfast means cereal' mindset most of your life, changing might be difficult, but it's well worth it. You'll enjoy not feeling bloated from the big carb hit, while the protein and intense nutrient content will ensure you won't feel hungry for hours afterwards.

For lunch

Salad – perfect for lunchtime. Add protein, including pulses, nuts or seeds, and really satisfy your hunger as well as your fibre and nutrient needs.

Adding cooked vegetables to salad gives extra variety and a different texture. Use cold leftovers from a previous meal or cook some fresh if you have time.

A time-saving salad hack

Prepare salads any time you're in the kitchen with the chopping board and knife. Store the chopped vegetables without dressing in an airtight container. Put wet veg (e.g. cucumber, tomatoes, avocado, cooked veg) on the bottom, leaves on top. Salad to go.

For dinner

Load up on non-starchy veg such as leafy greens, broccoli and cabbage, as well as pulses. Avoid starchy vegetables with dinner.

For snacks

Celery, carrot, capsicum, raw broccoli florets, leftover cooked vegetables – with or without cheese or hummus. Or leftover salad or cooked vegetables.

Super salad sprinkle

In a large glass screw-top jar, mix one third pepitas, one third sunflower seeds, and one third pine nuts. Add some chia seeds too if you like. Sprinkle over salads or cooked vegetables to add flavour, crunch and extra nutrients.

Store it in the fridge and use within three months (nuts, especially pine nuts, do eventually become rancid, but last longer in the fridge or freezer).

Get dressed

Make salad dressing yourself. Don't buy it, even if the label claims to be just oil and vinegar. Shop-bought varieties are generally high in sugar, processed oils and calories, as well as other additives and preservatives.

For example, a popular Australian brand of 'balsamic dressing' contains:

> *Water, Sunflower Oil [Antioxidant (320)], Balsamic Vinegar (15%) [wine vinegar, grape must, Preservative (224) (sulphites), Colour (150d)] Sugar, Lemon Juice Concentrate [Food Acid (330), preservative (223) (Sulphites)], White Vinegar, Salt, Garlic (0.7%) [Food acid (330)], Mineral Salts (332, 341, 508), Vegetable Gums (407, 410, 415 from Soy, 440), Red Bell Pepper, Parsley (0.03%).*

Phew! But at least they're honest.

Easy salad dressing (also delicious on cooked vegetables)

- Find a small glass jar with a well-fitting screw-on lid.

- Fill 1/3 of the jar with extra virgin olive oil.

- Add balsamic vinegar until the jar is 2/3 full. (***Avoid 'balsamic glaze'*** – it's vinegar mixed with a slug of sugar and other ingredients.)

- Add a generous amount of ground black pepper and a little salt.

- Shake well and use.

Keep it out on the kitchen bench or pantry; it doesn't need to be refrigerated and will last for weeks.

Experiment with taste – use different types of vinegar, or add a little lemon or lime juice, mixed herbs, chillies, or mustard.

Juicing

It's really popular, I know. But juicing is not necessarily good for us, and *it does not help us shed weight*.

Juicing removes fibre, or at best, pulverises it. So we get all the sugars and micronutrients in a concentrated form – far more than we'd be likely to have naturally. It takes three or four oranges, or half a celery, or half a kilo of carrots, to make just one glass of juice.

Removing the fibre means missing out on its benefits, which are essential for weight management. Fibre helps stabilise blood sugar and suppress appetite and it's also key to keeping gut biota healthy and happy. Juicing also means missing out on the act of chewing (Chapter 6 has more about why chewing is so important). And then there's the sugar and overall energy content. Juice (unless you're using *only* green vegetables) packs a significant carb hit. The result is a blood sugar spike and efficient conversion of excess energy to fat.

What about blenders instead of juicers?

A juicing machine extracts fibre, but blenders do not – the whole fruit or vegetable remains in the blender. Does this make it much better? ***Not if your goal is weight reduction.*** Blending (particularly in 'extreme' blenders) breaks down the food's cellular structure. Once the juice reaches your gut, there is not enough effective fibre remaining to slow down conversion of juice to glucose.

What's in it?

A glass of plain carrot juice contains about 30 g of sugar. In terms of vitamins and minerals, half a kilo of carrots is good for potassium and sodium, and a reasonable start for daily calcium and magnesium, but not for much else.

Juice from greens (e.g. celery, cucumber and kale) gives a better nutrient balance, without the sugar load. More than enough vitamin C, plus a high proportion of some essential minerals – calcium, iron, magnesium, phosphorus, potassium, sodium and zinc.

Juice from fresh oranges? Sugar at 41 g per glass. While high in vitamin C (five times more than the recommended daily intake), it is lower in most vitamins and minerals than vegetable juice.

If you do choose to juice, aim for mostly green vegetables to prevent blood sugar spikes. Add only small quantities of sweeter vegetables (e.g. carrots) and avoid fruit.

HABIT HELPERS – EAT MORE VEGETABLES

Meals means greens. Have non-starchy vegetables with every meal. When preparing a main meal, think 'salad *and* veg' (not salad *or* veg).

Veg first. Always serve vegetables first, and make sure they take up at least half the plate.

Know your starches. The main starchy vegetables are potato and sweet potato, sweet corn, parsnips and pumpkin. Think of starchy veg as grains, not greens. Although pulses contain starch, they're an important source of protein and fibre, so we don't include them as starchy veg.

Smarten them up. Home-made dressing – a simple olive oil and vinegar mix – goes beautifully with cooked vegetables as well as salad. A scatter of raw mixed seeds (e.g. pumpkin, chia and sunflower) adds interesting texture as well as healthy fats and protein.

REFLECTIONS

- How many serves of vegetables (*not counting* potatoes or pulses) do you have each day? A 'serve' is one packed cup of raw vegetables (e.g. salad), or ½ cup of cooked vegetables.

- How will you get more vegetables and a wider range of vegetables, especially greens, into your day? One of my favourites is roughly chopped kale, broccoli and green beans, fried with a little olive oil and salt and pepper in a very hot pan for about five minutes.

Plenty of protein

The short story on protein

Eat more protein. Protein is an essential tool for reducing weight while staying healthy and not feeling deprived. Everyone needs *at least* 1 g per kilo of body weight, per day, and more than this as we get older. To shed excess body fat, *aim for 1.2–1.5 g protein per kilo* of body weight.

Green zone: Eat more protein from high-quality, unprocessed or low-processed sources:

- fish and other seafood
- grass-fed meat and poultry, including chicken, turkey, kangaroo, beef and lamb
- eggs
- tofu or tempeh (unflavoured)
- pulses such as chickpeas, lentils, kidney beans, split peas
- cheese and yoghurt (dairy).

Amber zone: Eat less (be cautious with quantities) processed meat such as ham, bacon, sausages and patties, and processed vegetarian meat substitutes.

Red zone: Avoid protein products that are fried and/or processed with carbs, such as pies, sausage rolls, nuggets, and battered or crumbed foods.

Why protein?

We need to eat *enough protein every day*. We break down protein we eat into amino acids – building blocks we use for growing and repairing almost all our cells and body tissues, including muscles. We need 20 different types of amino acids, and while our body makes some of these itself, it cannot make them all: nine must come from our diet on a daily basis. These are known as the 'essential' amino acids.[19]

Eat protein to shed excess weight

Apart from being necessary for life, eating enough protein helps us reach and remain at our ideal weight.

The weight-management benefits of protein are well-established by research, which shows that eating protein:

---

[19]   The essential amino acids are histidine, isoleucine, leucine, lysine, methionine, phenylalanine, threonine, tryptophan and valine.

- reduces appetite and keeps us feeling fuller for longer, so we're less likely to feel hungry or overeat

- helps keep blood sugar low and stable, which in turn avoids laying down extra body fat

- develops muscles and helps prevent muscle loss. Apart from keeping us strong, muscle tissue uses more energy than fat tissue, so the more muscle we have, the faster we burn through excess energy and fat stores

- preserves muscle mass as we shed weight. If we reduce the amount we eat without making sure we're still getting enough daily protein, our body will take the protein it needs from our own muscles (including potentially our heart muscle)

- uses more energy to digest than either fat or carbs

- avoids the 'skinny-fat' problem. When we don't eat enough protein, we lose muscle mass and cannot regain muscle tone, regardless of how much exercise we do. You often see the result in people who have been 'dieting' in the wrong way for too long. They may not weigh much, but most of it is fat tissue, with very little muscle.

How much protein?

We need somewhere between 1–2 g of protein per kilogram of our body weight every day. For example, someone who weighs 80 kg needs at least 80 g of protein each day.

If our goal is to shed fat, then we need to *aim for the higher end of the range*, around 1.5 g per kilo of body weight every day (especially if we're older, or postmenopausal). Studies repeatedly show that diets with higher amounts of protein result in greater fat reduction than lower protein diets.

We need to distribute our protein intake across the day, because we can't effectively store it. Including a concentrated source of protein in at least three meals per day also helps stave off hunger. Studies from Australia's leading science agency, CSIRO, suggest we should be aiming for *20–30 g at each meal*.

> ### What's age got to do with it?
>
> As we age, a process called sarcopenia will stalk us. Sarcopenia is the gradual degeneration of muscle tissue, and it can happen whether we're lean or carrying extra body fat.
>
> We can protect ourselves from sarcopenia by increasing exercise, especially resistance exercise, and *eating more protein*.

Sources of protein

The 'grams of protein per kilo per day' recommendation means protein *in its pure form*. But not even a piece of steak is pure protein! To make sure we're eating enough, we need to know roughly how much protein is in different foods. We should also notice what makes up the remainder of the weight – is it fat, carbs, fibre or water?

The table below shows the *average* amount of protein in different types of food, as a percentage of the weight of the food. You only need a 'close enough' guide; precision isn't important here.

PROTEIN AS % OF TOTAL WEIGHT

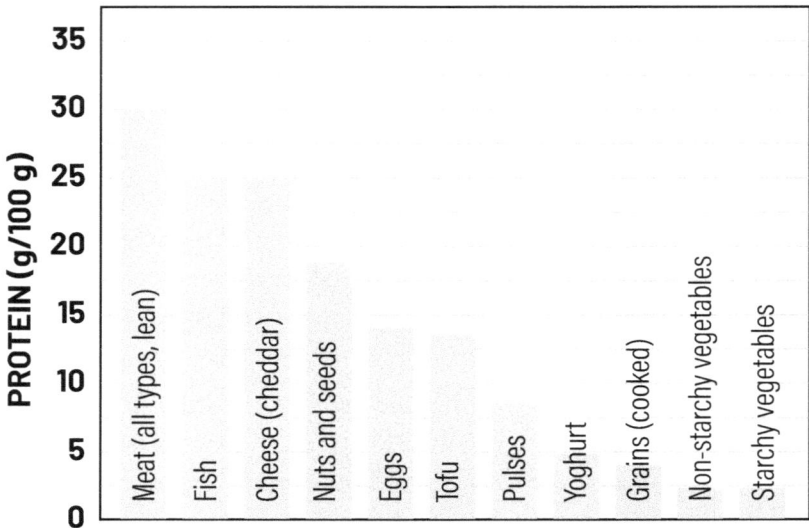

Meat in all forms is the highest source of protein by weight. Lean red and white meat, including poultry, has roughly 30 g protein per 100 g. The fattier the cut, the lower the protein content.

Fish has around 25 g protein per 100 g. Again, fat content matters, so a fatty fish such as salmon is lower in protein by weight than a leaner white fish.

All meat and fish, and most seafood, contain no carbs.[20]

Hard cheese also comes in at around 25 g per 100 g. The higher a cheese's fat content (e.g. brie) or water content (e.g. cottage cheese), the lower the protein will be by weight.

Nuts and seeds are just under 20 g protein per 100 g, with high fat content and a moderate amount of fibre.

Eggs and tofu are 10–15 g protein per 100 g. Tofu has no carbs and eggs have just a little. Eggs are about 9 g fat, while tofu varies, depending how it is made.

Pulses average about 7 g protein per 100 g when cooked. They're very low in fat and high in fibre, with a moderate amount of digestible carbs.

Yoghurt (unsweetened, dairy) has close to 5 g protein per 100 g. It also has about 5 g each of fat and carbs per 100 g. The protein content of dairy-free yoghurt varies widely between types and brands.

Cooked grains have just 3–4 g protein per 100 g. They're high in carbs with some fibre. Although often held up as good sources of meat-free protein, whole grains including ancient grains such as quinoa, freekeh and spelt only just scrape in as a source of protein, at around 15% of their energy value.[21] They are rich in fibre, vitamins and minerals, though, and well worth eating. White rice has the

---

[20]   Mussels, clams, oysters and octopus contain tiny amounts of carbs.

[21]   As protein, fat and carbs provide different amounts of energy (calories) per 100 g, protein as a proportion of energy value is different from protein by weight. The relative energy value provided by protein depends how much fat, carbs and water the food also contains.

least to offer nutritionally – truly empty carbs. Think of grains as mostly a *source of carbs, not protein*.

Vegetables are lowest in protein by weight (varying around 1–4 g), as they are mostly water and fibre, with minimal fat, and are low in calories overall. The World Health Organization's recommended 400 g of non-starchy vegetables per day provides about 10–15 g protein. Non-starchy vegetables are very low in carbs; starchy vegetables are high in carbs.

Working out how much protein is in your food

This book isn't about weighing food, so I'm not suggesting you need to make complex calculations about your protein intake (unless you're curious and that's your thing).

It's not necessary to know precisely how much protein is in everything you eat. Just get used to recognising good sources of protein – use the table in this section, or go to the Five for Life website for a list of food servings that provide around 20 g protein. The Food Standards Australia New Zealand (FSANZ) Australian Food Composition Database is an excellent resource, setting out the entire nutritional profile (including vitamins, minerals and trace elements) of thousands of different foods.[22]

Packaged food will show protein content in the label's nutrition information panel. Chapter 12 has more about using nutrition labels.

Best protein sources

The best protein sources are the ones you like and are comfortable with eating in the quantities you need them.

It's important to choose protein that is close to its natural state. Items like chicken nuggets, hotdogs, fish fingers, schnitzels and processed reconstituted ham, turkey, chicken and beef aren't our friends. It's not just the flavourings and preservatives in these

---

[22] https://www.foodstandards.gov.au/science/monitoringnutrients/afcd/Pages/foodsearch.aspx.

processed foods that makes them unhealthy – the crumbing, battering, vegetable oils and 'fillers' are fattening.

Canned pulses and fish are fine. For canned fish, make sure it's in pure olive oil or spring water.

Vegetarian and vegan sources of protein

Although animal products contain the highest amount of protein by both weight and energy value, it's not difficult to get plenty of protein from vegetable sources. Many of the world's cultures have large or even mostly vegetarian populations, so there are plenty of inspirational cuisines to get your ideas from. Have a look at Indian, Thai, Ethiopian, Korean and Mexican.

Most plant protein does not contain all nine essential amino acids in the quantities we need them; soy is the main exception. To make sure you get all these building blocks, mix up your protein sources through the day, including pulses, nuts and seeds, and some whole grains.

Vegetarian protein sources

Pulses – lentils, chickpeas, kidney beans, butter beans, broad beans, black beans, navy beans, white beans, cannellini beans, split peas and green peas.

Nuts – choose raw, unsalted nuts with the skin on. Try out activated nuts for a completely different taste and texture.

Seeds – chia, sunflower, pepita, pumpkin and sesame seeds (including tahini, the creamy paste made from ground sesame seeds).

Yoghurt and cheese – dairy-sourced yoghurt and cheese (especially cottage cheese) are good sources of protein. Non-dairy equivalents may not be as high in protein, and may contain other additives – check the labels.

Processed proteins – tofu and tempeh (both from soybeans) and seitan (wheat gluten) originated in Asian cultures and have been used for hundreds of years; these are the least processed of the processed proteins. Unflavoured, unfried versions do not include artificial additives or processed vegetable oil.

Other processed proteins, including mycoprotein derived from fungus (Quorn™), textured vegetable protein and many others, are usually heavily processed combinations of wheat, soy, peas and other pulses. Check the labels carefully, and avoid additives such as flavourings, sugar, colour, vegetable oil (unless it specifies olive oil) and ingredients you don't recognise. In my experience, modern processed proteins are mostly interesting only for novelty value.

Count the other macronutrients too

The food we eat for protein generally contains some fat and carbs, too.

- If pulses are your main protein source, remember to also consider them in your overall daily carb intake.

- Nuts provide protein but are also high in fat. Ditto for most cheese, except cottage cheese, which is low in fat and carbs, and high in protein.

- Whole grains provide some protein but are mostly carbs.

HABIT HELPERS – EAT PLENTY OF PROTEIN

Work it out. Calculate how much protein you need per day, and decide, roughly, how you'll get it.

Spread it around. Distribute your protein across the day, around 20–30 g in each main meal. Very roughly, that's about

100 g (uncooked) of meat or fish, or about 70–80 g once cooked. The Five for Life website has examples of 20 g serves of protein from both animal and plant sources.

Quick and easy. Feeling hungry? Add protein – a simple, protein-based meal or snack like a boiled egg, a can of fish, a tub of plain yoghurt or cottage cheese, a piece of steamed chicken or fish, or some tofu.

Get out of the rut. Go online if you're out of ideas. There are many websites with suggestions for 'top ten' healthy protein sources and meal ideas – for vegans, vegetarians and meat-eaters.

REFLECTIONS

- What is the *minimum* amount of protein you need to aim for each day? Calculate your weight, in kilograms, multiplied by 1.2 g of protein = minimum grams of protein for shedding body fat.

- What are your main sources of protein, and how much of those foods do you need each day to get your recommended minimum protein?

  Remember – protein only makes up part of any food type, so for example 100 g chicken doesn't equal 100 g protein. The highest protein content food is meat (including poultry), at around 25–35 g per 100 g.

- What changes will you make to be sure to get enough protein, every day?

Sufficient 'good' fat

The short story on fats

The most important thing about fats is to have them natural, not processed.

Green zone: Eat most

- raw nuts and seeds

- avocados

- fish, such as salmon, sardines and mackerel

- cold-pressed plant oils, such as virgin olive oil, macadamia oil and avocado oil.

Amber zone: Eat moderately (be cautious with quantities)

- cold-pressed coconut oil and cocoa butter

- animal fat close to its natural state – e.g. in unprocessed meat, milk, butter, cream and cheese.

Red zone: Avoid

Avoid all trans fats and processed fats. These are contained in:

- fast food and most takeaway, particularly anything deep-fried

- commercially made baked goods – e.g. pastries, popcorn, pizza, pies, croissants and desserts

- processed vegetable oils and products containing these oils – e.g. margarine and manufactured sauces, mayonnaise and salad dressings, many baked goods and other manufactured goods

- processed food that's high in saturated fat – e.g. processed meat products including nuggets, canned luncheon meat and most commercially made sausages.

Why fat?

Don't be frightened of fat – it's not a dirty word.

We need to eat fat for a whole range of reasons:

- So our body can access and use fat-soluble compounds, including vitamins A, D, E and K.
- To provide us with essential fatty acids that our body can't produce on its own (Omega-6 and Omega-3).
- To protect our heart, and protect our brain from memory loss and dementia *(fats from plants and fish only)*.
- To improve our skin and prevent inflammatory conditions like eczema.
- To prevent and reduce symptoms of depression and other mood disorders *(mainly Omega-3 fatty acids)*.

Fat we eat vs. fat we store in our body

Fat we eat is called 'dietary fat'. It's not the same as the fat we store in our body (referred to as body fat, adipose tissue or fat cells). Dietary fat does not proceed directly to be stored in our own fat cells. *Eating fat doesn't 'make you fat'.*

Dietary fat is part of our overall energy intake, just like the energy we get from carbs and protein. Our body uses what it can in the hours after we eat, but if we consume more than we need, the excess is eventually converted into a type of fat (triglycerides) and stored in our fat cells.

How much fat?

The best research tells us that ***at least 30%*** of our daily energy intake (calories) should be from fat.[23] This means somewhere ***between 50 and 100 g of fat per day***, depending on your overall energy intake.

---

[23] The Australian Dietary Guidelines and Nutrient Reference Values for Australia and New Zealand (Fats: Total fat and fatty acids) recommend 20–35%, but these do not reflect more recent research. A moderate-fat Mediterranean diet, well known for its health benefits, is about 35–45% fat, with much of that coming from olive oil. A keto diet will be considerably higher in fat.

Some sources of high-quality dietary fat

- a small piece of Atlantic salmon (100 g) – 19 g of fat
- a small handful of almonds (30 g or 25 nuts) – 15 g of fat
- a tablespoon of olive oil (about 15 ml) – 14 g of fat
- half an avocado (about 80 g) – 10 g of fat
- a glass of full-fat milk (250 ml) – 9 g of fat.

It's worth remembering that because fat is very dense in energy (nearly twice as much energy per gram as protein or carbs), it's easy to overeat and this can undermine our weight goals. Unless you're on a keto diet, do keep an eye on your intake. As you can see from the examples, it doesn't take much to get to 50 g.

Different types of fats

We eat three types of fat:

- *Unsaturated fats.* Avocados, olives, nuts and seeds, and seafood and eggs, are high in unsaturated fats. There are two types – *monounsaturated* (the richest source is olive oil) and *polyunsaturated* (Omega-3 and Omega-6 essential fatty acids). These are found mostly in nuts, seeds and fish, but also in smaller amounts in grass-fed meat, and eggs from free range pastured hens.

- *Saturated fats.* The highest concentration of saturated fats is in the flesh of animals, and in animal products – milk, cream, butter, cheese and eggs.[24] Coconut, palm and cocoa oil are also mostly saturated fat.

- *Trans fats.* Very small amounts of trans fats occur naturally in animal products. Mostly, however, trans fats are manufactured by adding hydrogen to plant oils to make them solid at room temperature. Trans fats are frequently used in deep-frying, and

---

[24] Eggs are about 50% unsaturated and 50% saturated fat.

in packaged baked goods such as cakes, biscuits and pastries. Trans fats are dangerous for our health.

Most fat-containing food has a mix of the different types of fats, but is higher in one type than another.

Best fat sources – fats in their natural state

Get *most* of your fat from **plants and fish in their natural state**: oily fish such as salmon and mackerel, raw nuts and seeds, avocados and olives. Vegetable oils that are cold-pressed and unrefined are also good sources of fat. Extra virgin olive oil and avocado oil are the best of these; coconut oil is another good source. 'Cold-pressed' oils are produced by simply forcing oil out of the nut or seed through pressure, without altering the natural structure or nutrient value of the oil.

It's perfectly fine to have *some* fat from **animal sources** – provided it's natural or low-processed, such as the fat in meat and eggs, and in animal products like butter, milk, cream and cheese.

But isn't saturated fat 'bad'?

Debate continues to rage over the health status of saturated fats, which are mostly found in animal products, but also in coconut and palm oil. There are many different types of saturated fats, and they function in different ways. Different foods contain varying quantities of different types of fat, as well as other nutrients. No good-quality studies have yet drilled down into the effects of different types of saturated fats in the context of the overall 'food matrix' (the physical and chemical properties of whole foods) and overall diets.

The best evidence at the moment suggests that saturated fat does not increase the incidence of heart disease. However, it is clear that saturated fat *in processed food* should be avoided, as it contains unhealthy chemical compounds. Whole-fat dairy, unprocessed meat and dark chocolate can be healthy sources of fat provided they're eaten as part of a diet that is also *low in refined and starchy carbs and sugar.* In a large study of nearly 200,000 participants followed for more than 10 years, and to nobody's surprise, the diet least associated with death from any cause was high in fibre and monounsaturated fats, moderate in starch and protein, and low in saturated fats, polyunsaturated fats and sugar.[25]

Even though saturated fat in its natural state isn't necessarily 'bad', monounsaturated fats (such as olive oil) and Omega-3 and Omega-6 in their natural state have greater health benefits.

In particular, studies show monounsaturated fats play an important role in regulating weight, whereas saturated fats do not. This means we're better off getting the bulk of our fat from fish, raw nuts and seeds, avocados and cold-pressed vegetable oil, especially olive oil. And going easy on the cheese, butter and cream.

The Omega-6 question

The essential fatty acids Omega-3 and Omega-6 are often referred to as 'good fats', as they have many health benefits.

In the right balance, it's true that these fats are beneficial. But we need to balance our intake so that for every unit of Omega-3, we have between one and four units of Omega-6. This was the natural state of our diet until just over 100 years ago. These days, we eat far too much Omega-6 (typically more than 1:10; even up to 1:20), throwing this delicate ratio right out of whack. Why? Because we have reduced our intake of saturated fat (we were told that butter and eggs are bad for us) and largely replaced it with processed vegetable oils like sunflower, corn, soy and canola. These oils are very high in Omega-6, and widely used in manufactured food. It's difficult to avoid Omega-6.

Is this a problem? In short, most likely yes. There is increasing evidence to suggest that having too much Omega-6 in the form of processed vegetable oils may be the culprit for a range of diseases including obesity and coronary heart disease. While studies are

---

[25] Ho (2020) Associations of fat and carbohydrate intake with cardiovascular disease and mortality: prospective cohort study of UK Biobank participants.

inconsistent, the high Omega-6 content of many refined vegetable oils links them with chronic inflammation and associated diseases. The refining process also damages the oils, including by reducing their nutritional content. The section below on 'fats to avoid' looks more closely at processed vegetable oils.

It's almost impossible to correct our Omega-6:3 balance by simply eating more Omega-3 (e.g. oily fish or supplements). Focus instead on reducing intake of processed vegetable oils and products containing them.

What's up with coconut oil?

Coconut oil used to be labelled 'wholly bad' because it's mainly saturated fat. But now we know that saturated fats aren't necessarily bad, where does that leave coconut oil?

The chemical structure of coconut oil is different from other saturated fats, in ways that may have specific health benefits, although studies are mixed.[26] The main concern is that coconut oil raises LDL ('bad') cholesterol. While it also raises HDL ('good') cholesterol, this isn't enough to maintain the right ratio of LDL to HDL.

My advice is – by all means use coconut oil (I do, as it's delicious and great for cooking), but don't eat it by the tablespoon, and make sure to use *more* of the unsaturated, unprocessed plant oils, especially olive oil.

Fats to avoid

Avoid any fat that is not in its natural, or close-to-natural, form. So – *avoid manufactured trans fats and highly processed vegetable oils*.

---

[26] Coconut oil is a blend of short and medium-chain fatty acids (MCTs), unlike other saturated fats. While some studies have shown that humans decrease their food intake when they have a diet rich in MCTs, other studies have shown that the effect only lasts for a single meal, and the body adapts to MCTs if they are eaten regularly. Coconut oil is about 50% MCT, but there's not much evidence that we get direct MCT benefits from eating coconut oil.

Trans fats

Trans fats increase the risk of heart disease by raising LDL cholesterol and lowering HDL cholesterol. Some human and animal research also links trans fats to insulin resistance and increased abdominal fat.

Trans fats are created when liquid oils are processed by adding hydrogen to solidify them for use in baking and for spreads (hydrogenated vegetable oils). Trans fats are also formed when oils or fats are repeatedly heated at very high temperatures, such as when they're used in deep-frying, or during the processing treatment of refined vegetable oils.[27]

Trans fats extend shelf-life of manufactured foods, so they're often used in processed food and manufactured baked goods. They're also frequently used in deep-fryers. A recent study comparing trans fat content of various manufactured items found that most of the Australian products tested were significantly higher in trans fats than equivalent products in Canada, UK, Netherlands and Malaysia.[28]

Trans fats don't have to be included on the nutrition label of Australian food, but we can tell by checking the ingredients list: 'vegetable fat' or 'partially hydrogenated vegetable oil' means the product contains trans fats.

The best way to avoid trans fats is to:

- avoid fried food, including pre-fried frozen foods such as chips, nuggets and spring rolls

- avoid commercially made baked foods such as cakes, biscuits, pastries, donuts and pies

- avoid packaged food that lists 'partially hydrogenated vegetable oil' or 'vegetable fat' as an ingredient.

---

[27] Small amounts of *natural* trans fats occur in meat and dairy from ruminants (cows, sheep and goats), but these are of no concern.

[28] Wu (2017) Levels of trans fats in the food supply and population consumption in Australia: an Expert Commentary for The National Heart Foundation of Australia.

Palm oil

Palm oil is often used as a substitute for trans fats, because it is naturally solid at room temperature. Although palm oil is better for your health than trans fats, it's no good for the planet.

Restrictions on the use of trans fats in the US since 2018 have resulted in a dramatic increase in demand for palm oil. Palms grow in tropical places, so vast areas of rainforest are cleared every year to make way for bigger palm plantations. The result is a tragic acceleration of forest clearance, and death of orangutans, tigers and other species who called those forests home.

Highly processed vegetable oils

Highly processed vegetable oils include canola, sunflower, corn and soybean oils.

Processed (or 'refined') oil production involves extracting oil from seeds or kernels using chemical solvents and very high temperatures, then bleaching and deodorising it. Vegetable oils are also often treated with hydrogen, creating trans fats. The result of all this processing is a damaged oil that is linked to inflammatory conditions, including obesity. It's high in Omega-6, and low or absent in Omega-3 and other nutrients.

Avoiding highly processed vegetable oil means first recognising where it is. And it's in a lot of places.

Vegetable oil improves the flavour, texture and shelf-life of manufactured goods and it's cheap, so a huge range of manufactured items use it, including margarine and vegetable shortening, dips, cakes, biscuits, pastries, chips and snack foods – even food we might think is a healthier choice, such as muesli bars. Always check the ingredients list of packaged food. 'Vegetable oil' or 'vegetable fat' means the product contains highly processed seed or bean oil. If the oil has been hydrogenated, it will also contain trans fats.

As processed vegetable oil is inexpensive, it's the oil of choice in commercial food outlets and many cafes and restaurants. Avoid takeaway and limit the amount of restaurant food you have.

Deep-fried food

Deep-fried food combines everything that's 'bad' about fats, and *it's an 'almost never' food*. The oil used will be processed vegetable oil, it will have been heated to high temperatures, and will most likely have been reheated a number of times. Deep-fried stuff is also generally very high in carbs – chips and battered things. This takes you straight to the danger zone – carbs prepared with fat and added sugar and/or salt.

Nuts – are they all they're cracked up to be?

Yes! Nuts are high in 'good' fats, high in fibre, and extraordinarily nutritious. Have them raw and unsalted, and remember that they're also high in calories. Be sparing with brazils (limit of one or two per day) due to their significant selenium content.

Naked nuts are nicest

Nuts are often sold as roasted and/or salted. Sometimes they're presented (tantalisingly) as covered in both sugar and salt (honey-caramelised cashews, anyone?), luring us into a dangerously moreish combination of fat, sugar and salt. Nuts like this won't help you reach your best weight.

- *Eat them raw.* When nuts are roasted, they lose some of their health benefits. Some of the natural fats and other nutrients are damaged or destroyed, and harmful chemicals are created if nuts are roasted at high temperatures.

- *Unsalted.* Too much salt is linked to high blood pressure and the diseases associated with that, and most Australians eat nearly twice as much salt as we need to. Also – salted nuts are almost always roasted first, negating many of the benefits of nuts.

- *Skin-on.* The skin of nuts (especially almonds and hazelnuts) contains fibre and substances called polyphenols, one of the many health-giving properties of nuts. Eat them skin-on.

What about activated nuts?

Activated nuts have been soaked in water, then dried out at low temperatures, retaining all nutrients and the quality of the fats. They have a deliciously different flavour from raw or roasted nuts. Be aware of added salt, though, as activated nuts have generally been soaked in salt water, and are sometimes coated in salt or flavouring during the drying process.

It's been claimed that activating nuts makes their minerals more easily absorbed, because the soaking removes compounds known as phytates, but the evidence doesn't support this idea. Only two studies seem to have been conducted: one, in 2018, found that almonds were *higher* in phytates when soaked, than not.[29] The other (2020) found that soaked nuts did on average have slightly lower phytate levels, but that the activation process reduces mineral levels overall, meaning that there was no net benefit.[30]

High in calories

Nuts are full of good fats, but this means they're 'energy dense' – they are high in calories.

But we aren't counting calories, right? Right. However, it's easy to overdo nuts. They're extremely tasty, and don't take up much physical room in our stomach. Because of this, we can eat a lot before our stomach-brain connection has time to register 'enough'. And if our stomach is used to holding large quantities before it tells our brain it's full, by the time that happens we've eaten too many nuts. Because fat is high in calories, this is when the 'calories-in' part of the equation does actually matter.[31]

---

[29] Taylor (2018) The effects of 'activating' almonds on consumer acceptance and gastrointestinal tolerance.

[30] Kumari (2020) Does 'activating' nuts affect nutrient bioavailability?

[31] If you follow a ketogenic diet with daily carbs below 50 g, calories from fat are not an issue, but the carb content might be – some nuts contain more carbs than others.

Treat yourself to one small cupped handful of raw, unflavoured nuts every day. As our hands tend to be roughly proportional in size to the rest of our frame, this is likely to be the right amount for you.

Cooking with oils

Cooking plant or animal oils at high temperatures causes them to break down, decreasing the amount of antioxidants and damaging more fragile oils such as Omega-3. If oils are heated to smoking point, they also release harmful free radicals and other compounds. Avoid overheating oils, including in stir-fry. Coconut and olive oil are good choices for stir-fry, as they can handle higher cooking temperatures before breaking down. Alternatively, use a high-quality non-stick pan and add oil shortly before you finish cooking.

Limit how much you shallow or deep-fry food. Treat it as a 'now and then' event (I'm talking *monthly, not daily or weekly*). Use a fat that can handle higher temperatures before it creates trans-fatty acids or breaks down to release free radicals – coconut, olive or avocado oil are good ones. Don't re-use cooking oil. The more it's heated, the more damaging it becomes.

HABIT HELPERS – EAT SUFFICIENT GOOD FAT

Keep it natural. Natural and unprocessed is always best.

Have it home-made. The best way to know what types of fats are in the food you eat is to make it yourself.

Fear of frying. Avoid fried food, especially if it's been in a deep-fryer, or the supermarket fridge/freezer.

Clear it out. Check your cupboards and fridge. Keep your cold-pressed olive, macadamia, avocado, or coconut oils (check they're within use-by dates). Throw out oil that is not cold pressed, as heavily processed oils are a risk to your health. Check for food that contains 'vegetable oil' as a listed ingredient. Limit how often you eat it, and avoid buying more.

Read up. Read labels of packaged food – look for 'vegetable oil', 'vegetable fat', 'partially hydrogenated vegetable oil' and 'vegetable shortening'. Put it back on the shelf.

REFLECTIONS

- What are your favourite sources of high-quality, natural plant-based fats? How can you replace processed fats and animal fats with more of these?

- How often do you have raw, unsalted nuts? Which are your favourites, and what changes will you make to eat more nuts?

- How often do you have food that has been deep-fried? What will you do to reduce that?

- How often do you have commercially made baked goods (cakes, biscuits, or pastry-cased things), and what will you do to reduce the amount you have?

The right carbs

The short story on carbs

All starches, all sugars (including natural sugar in fruit, milk, and some vegetables) and all fibre are carbs. That's why carbs can feel confusing. In Five for Life, the carb question is simplified by using a traffic light system:

Green zone: Eat plenty

- greens and colourful, non-starchy vegetables
- pulses (e.g. chickpeas, lentils, kidney beans)

Amber zone: Eat moderately (be cautious with quantities)

- milk and yoghurt (plain and unsweetened)
- starchy vegetables (potato, sweet potato, sweet corn, parsnip and pumpkin)
- fruit (whole, not juiced)
- whole grains

Red zone: Eat least

- refined sugar
- refined starches (e.g. rice, flour and foods made of rice or flour)
- danger zone food – processed carbs with fat and flavouring.

Limiting red zone carbs is essential to reaching and staying at your happy weight.

Why carbohydrates?

Carbs are a big topic for healthy eating, because carbs as a category means *all starches, all sugars, and all types of fibre*. As fibre provides very little energy, 'carbs' in this book means starches and sugars (if I mean fibre, I'll say so).

Carbs are a quick energy source, as they're rapidly converted into glucose that we can use immediately for energy. But if we're not using that fuel in the next couple of hours, it gets easily stored, mostly in the form of body fat. The more carbs we eat in one sitting, the more likely we'll be storing body fat from that meal or snack.

Some high-carb foods are healthy *in the right amount*. These are the 'whole foods' – plants close to their natural state, including pulses, fruit, starchy vegetables and whole grains. Naturally rich in vitamins, minerals and fibre, they may include some protein and a little fat.

On the other hand, foods high in processed, refined carbs (including sugar and flour) offer almost no other nutrients, just 'empty' calories. They're poor quality, and essentially a waste of space.

Processed carbs are also often prepared in a way that makes us more likely to crave them: as sugar or starch laced with fat and flavourings. These are the *red zone carbs, and they include danger zone food.* These types of carbs are implicated in addictive-like eating behaviours and cravings, and are a major cause of over-eating, overweight, and the diseases and metabolic disorders that go with those.

Eat natural, not processed, especially when it comes to carbs.

Sources of carbs

All plants contain carbs – sugars, starches and fibres – in different quantities. The *only* animal-based foods that contain relevant amounts of carbs are milk and yoghurt (which contain sugar in the form of lactose)[32] and honey.

Fibre is the only type of carb that we don't digest enough of to generate significant energy (glucose). Although it doesn't provide energy, fibre is an incredibly important part of our diet. More on fibre later in this chapter.

Some foods are pure carbs (e.g. table sugar, made from refined sugar cane), but mostly, foods that we categorise as carbs also contains some other nutrients – perhaps a little protein or fat, and some vitamins and minerals. Some carb foods contain quite significant amounts of protein; these are pulses and legumes, and to a lesser extent, milk and yoghurt.

---

[32] Lactose-free milk replaces lactose with other sugars: glucose and galactose. Butter, cream and cheese normally have only very little lactose, due to their high fat and (for cheese) protein content.

THE TRAFFIC LIGHT TABLE FOR CARBS

GREEN ZONE (eat most)	**Non-starchy vegetables** E.g. all salad leaves, tomatoes, capsicum, cucumber and other salad vegetables, broccoli, cabbage, zucchini, cauliflower, leafy greens. Most non-starchy veg are less than 50% carbs by energy. **Pulses** E.g. chickpeas, lentils, kidney beans, black beans, butter beans and split peas. Because of their high protein content, pulses also count as a protein food.
AMBER ZONE (limit quantities)	**Starchy vegetables** The main ones are potatoes, sweet potatoes, sweet corn, parsnip, pumpkin, beetroot and carrots. **Fruit** Have up to two serves/day of whole fruit (not juice) until you reach your ideal weight. All your vitamins, minerals and fibre can come from vegetables, without the sugar. Choose mostly lower-sugar fruit – berries, kiwifruit, grapefruit, orange and watermelon. Once at your target weight, widen your fruit choices again but take care with quantities. **Whole grains and wholegrain products** E.g. unprocessed quinoa, oats, barley, spelt, buckwheat and wild or brown rice, and small quantities of pasta or bread made with wholegrain flour. **Yoghurt and milk** Unsweetened, unflavoured. Take care with milk, as it raises blood sugar rapidly.

RED ZONE (avoid)

Sugar

Sugar in all its forms. Cane sugar, organic raw sugar, honey, agave nectar, maple syrup and coconut sugar are all sugar. Sweets, lollies, jams and marmalades, syrups and sauces.

Beware of sugar in drinks too – soft drinks, flavoured milk and fruit juice (including 'no added sugar' juice, as it's still packed with fruit sugar).

Refined grains

White rice is the main refined grain we commonly eat as-is. Wheat, rice, corn and other grains are usually refined and processed to make flour.

Refined-grain products (including gluten-free)

Any products made with refined flour, e.g. bread, pasta, cake, biscuits, breakfast cereals.

Yoghurt and milk

Flavoured or sweetened.

DANGER ZONE

Processed starchy carbs prepared with fat and either or both sugar and salt

E.g. pizza, chips, pies and savoury snack food (potato crisps and soy chips), cakes, biscuits, pastries, donuts, desserts and sweet snack food including confectionery.

A word about potatoes...

Potatoes are an 'amber' carb, so they're high quality, right?

Sort of. But calorie for calorie, potatoes have two to three times more carbs than non-starchy vegetables – potatoes are pretty much all starch. They also have a high glycaemic index, less than half the protein of many other vegetables, and significantly fewer vitamins and minerals (especially if you eat them with the skin off).

The starch in warm or hot cooked potatoes raises blood sugar very quickly, loading our body with glucose it can't use straight away – so it gets stored as fat. Interestingly, cooked potato, *when cold*, is higher in resistant starch, which our body treats more like fibre.

Potatoes are often prepared with oil – roasted, deep-fried or mashed with butter, milk or cream – and seasoned with salt. At that point they become hyper-flavoursome and therefore too easy to overeat.

Limit potatoes, they aren't worth it. Fill up on other vegetables. If you're after something to roast, try carrots, pumpkin, beetroot or swede. They're lower in starch and generally higher in minerals. Cauliflower and brussels sprouts are also delicious roasted, and have no starch.

Know your breads and pastas

Bread and pasta made with refined-grain flour have limited nutritional value, and will contribute to weight gain. They're really just filler food.

Bread and pasta that are high in *wholegrain flour* can be counted as amber zone carbs. Fine to eat in limited quantities.

How do you know if bread or pasta includes enough whole grain? First, check the label. If it's high in whole grain, it will say so, because it's something to be proud of. If the label just says 'contains' whole wheat, whole grain, oats etc, these ingredients will be present in some quantity, along with refined (red zone) flours. The words *'enriched flour'* and *'wheat flour'* never mean whole grain.

Good-quality bread is heavy and dense, made with wholegrain flours. It's also preferably sourdough, which has been fermented and benefits your gut microbiome. It's not fluffy and sweet, and it's not called 'sandwich bread'. Good-quality bread is more expensive than bread made of refined flours, but you won't be eating much.

A growing selection of ultra-low-carb bread is appearing in supermarkets. It tends to be highly processed and include synthetically made fibres and other ingredients to give a bread-like texture. In my view, good-quality, naturally produced sourdough is still a better choice. Remember that 'low carb' isn't your ultimate goal; rather, it's good, low-processed food in the right quantities. If you're interested in trying ultra-low-carb bread, look for one with the fewest ingredients, a good amount of whole seeds and natural fibre such as psyllium.

For pasta – there are lots of alternatives to refined wheat. Pasta from buckwheat, chickpea, lentil or whole spelt flour is minimally processed and behaves like a heavier version of white pasta, with the benefit of extra protein. Or go for something entirely different, such as noodles made from the konjac plant (sometimes called shirataki noodles). They're much finer than pasta, a bit like thin rice noodles, with almost no carbs.

The glycaemic index

It does help to know a bit about the glycaemic index (GI), but don't get too hung up about it.

The GI is a measurement of *how easy* it is for our body to turn different carbs into glucose. The GI scale runs from 1 (lowest) to 100 (highest). High-GI carbs raise our blood sugar rapidly, which is useful if you're an athlete about to sprint, but otherwise not so good. Energy not being used in the next couple of hours, or replenishing glycogen, will be stored as body fat.

Dietary fat and protein do not raise our blood sugar. This means that the GI of foods that are a mix of carbs, fat and protein is lower than the GI of a pure carb, or mainly carb food. A chocolate biscuit, for example (high in fat), has a much lower GI than a bag of jelly snakes (no fat or protein).

The main high-GI foods to look out for are the usual suspects – sugar, potatoes and processed starches (bread, rice and foods made from processed flour).

Appendix B has more detail on the GI if you're interested, but the key points are:

- All green zone carbs have a low or very low GI.

- Amber zone carbs (including whole grains and fruit) have a higher GI than green zone, while red zone carbs generally have very high GI.

- Just because it's low GI doesn't mean it's 'good for you'. Junk food can be low GI if it's also high in fat (*the sly GI!*).

- GI of some amber and red zone carbs can be reduced a little, by changing the way they're prepared (more detail in the Appendix).

How much?

Australians generally eat far too many carbs, especially the wrong sort, and it's the main reason more than two out of three of us are not a safe weight. Why? Not because we're bad, stupid or lazy, but because low-quality carbs are all around us, and we're used to them. They're cheap, convenient, ubiquitous and heavily advertised.

Even diets we've been told are reasonably healthy are too high in carbs: think cereal or toast for breakfast along with a milky coffee; sweet or savoury biscuits mid-morning with your flat white; a sandwich or wrap and fruit juice for lunch; a muesli bar for that mid-afternoon slump; and pasta, potato bake or rice with dinner.

We've *just got into the habit* of eating too many carbs.

There is increasingly solid evidence that reducing carbs in our diet is an effective and safe way to shed excess body fat, and that reducing to extremely low levels (ketogenic diet) achieves rapid fat reduction and may even be able to reverse metabolic syndrome and type 2 diabetes. However, a ketogenic diet can be difficult to maintain, and unless you take care to include sufficient highly nutritious vegetables, there is a risk of not getting enough fibre, vitamins and minerals on a daily basis. Ketogenic diets aren't suitable during pregnancy or breastfeeding, or for people with various health issues including liver or kidney concerns. If you're interested in trying a ketogenic diet, seek the guidance of a nutritionist or dietitian.

I recommend a medium- to low-carb diet (30–45% of total daily energy) for sustainable weight reduction, with an upper limit of around 150 g (women and smaller adults) or 200 g (men and larger adults) per day.[33] All but the odd gram or two should be coming from the green and amber zones. No need to starve either – reducing carbs while eating more protein and high-quality fats helps dampen appetite, by regulating our appetite-related hormones. Eating more protein also helps to ensure we maintain our lean muscle mass and don't feel deprived of food.

Apart from reducing daily carbs, it's also important not to eat too many in one sitting. Approximately 15 g of carbs (that's about one slice of bread, a small banana or a small potato) raises blood glucose levels high enough that we release insulin to move that glucose into cells for energy – and ultimately into fat cells for storage, if we don't need energy right away. Keeping carb content low (30–40 g) each time we eat, and also avoiding high-GI carbs, helps avoid excess blood glucose and the resulting fat storage.

Estimating carb intake

Carb-containing food isn't 100% carbs (unless it's pure sugar), so you need to make some rough calculations to estimate carb intake.

As a broad rule of thumb:

- Non-starchy veg have negligible carbs by weight, so don't bother to count them.

- Pulses, fruit and starchy vegetables are about 10–20% carbs by weight.

---

[33] If you want to know exactly how much energy (total calories) you need for your particular height, current and desired weight and activity level, online calculators are available, e.g. https://www.nrv.gov.au/dietary-energy or https://www.eatforhealth.gov.au/webform/daily-energy-requirements-calculator.

- Cooked pasta, rice and bread average 30–45% carbs by weight.

- Whole grains are around 50–65% carbs by dry weight (but processed grain flour, the main ingredient in bread, cake and biscuits, is about 75–85% carbs by dry weight).

If it's packaged, use the nutrition label. Food labels in Australia must state carbs as grams per 100 g, as well as grams per serve.

Check the serving size. Be wary – manufacturers of snack food often understate the serving size, hiding the true carb content. For example, potato crisps are usually sold as a 25 g serving size – which is *about nine chips*. So while a small bag (100 g) can claim only 14 g of carbs per serve, will you really share this small bag with three other people, or only eat a quarter of it?

If it's not packaged… it's more complicated, but gets simpler with practice. You can get a carb-counter app for your phone for accuracy if you like. Many people with diabetes use these to get through their daily lives.

Example – carbs in unpackaged food

Sandwich – A small–medium bread roll has about 32 g of high-GI carbs, before having anything with it. Best to choose something else.

Salad – A cup of cooked quinoa contains 16 g of low-GI carbs. Add a source of protein, avocado, sun-dried tomatoes, cucumber, capsicum, broccoli florets and some crumbled feta cheese… and you've got a delicious, filling meal still barely over 18 g of high-quality carbs.

Fruit – A medium Jonathan apple, half a mango or a cup of cherries has around 20 g of carbs. A cup of grapes, 22 g. Lower carb options are a medium orange, or a cup of blueberries or chopped watermelon, at about 13 g of carbs.

Carb 'tolerance' levels

Some people can handle more carbs than others without gaining body fat. We are all different, and due to a genetic or metabolic difference, some people are able to eat more carbs than others without adverse effect. But these people tend to be the exception – most people, me included, can't handle high levels of carbs (particularly poor-quality carbs) safely.

How to do it

Meal-building

The easiest way to get proportions right without weighing things is simply to focus each meal on getting plenty of good-quality, unprocessed protein and a little fat, along with a heap of green zone vegetables (non-starchy vegetables and pulses). Small amounts of fruit, starchy vegetables or whole grains are optional, and avoid having these at your last meal for the day.

Take out added sugar

Remove obvious sugar from your diet – in tea and coffee, and spread on bread. And no more soft drinks, sports drinks, flavoured milk or fruit juice. Cutting down added sugar can be difficult; the next section gets into that in more detail.

Go for quality

Choose high-quality carbs. Go for mostly green zone (non-starchy vegetables and pulses) and some amber zone (starchy vegetables, whole grains or lower-sugar fruit). Avoid red zone and danger zone carbs.

Download the Traffic Light Table for Carbs from the Five for Life website and keep it handy.

Keep an eye on quantity

Keep carbs below 30–40 g per meal. This means:

- non-starchy vegetables – any quantity, as their carb content is extremely low
- sweeter or starchy vegetables, whole grains or lower-sugar fruit – up to ¾ cup in total; for example:
  - » potatoes, sweet potatoes, sweet corn, parsnips, pumpkins and beetroot, or peas and carrot
  - » oats, quinoa, and wild or brown rice
  - » berries, citrus or watermelon
- pulses (e.g. chickpeas, kidney beans, lentils) – up to 1 cup (or 1½ cups if this is your main source of protein in the meal; beware of total carbs if you're combining pulses with starchy vegetables).

Even small amounts of red zone or danger zone carbs will quickly bring you over the 40 g threshold, with little or no nutritional benefit.

Watch the clock

Studies show that our body prefers to burn carbs as fuel in the first part of the day, so having most of our daily carbs before about 3 pm allows us to get the most out of our overnight fat-burning fast.

Push back on conditioning

Many (perhaps most) of us have been brought up assuming that a 'balanced meal' involves carbs. A meal *with* bread, pasta, potatoes, rice or other grains. Remember the old 'food pyramid' for supposedly healthy eating? The one we're probably most used to seeing was published by the US Department of Agriculture in 1992 (clue – support grain farmers). It recommended we should be eating at least six and *up to 11 serves per day* of bread, cereal, rice and pasta – and that advice is still often repeated today, in spite of what we know about these types of carbs.

We're heavily conditioned to expect to see carbs on our plate, and it's time to resist that. A protein source with some high-quality fat and plenty of vegetables *is a balanced meal.*

Fibre – essential to healthy weight

The short story? Eat more fibre to help reduce weight.

There's far more to fibre than just keeping our bowels moving regularly. High-fibre diets are *strongly associated with both weight reduction and maintenance of healthy weight,* but most of us aren't having enough (which is 28–38 g per day).[34]

Fibre:

- helps us feel fuller for longer, as it's bulky and fills the stomach

- helps keep blood sugar and energy levels stable. Fibre helps slow down the release of glucose into our bloodstream from the carbs we eat, reducing blood sugar spikes, and the amount of excess energy to be stored as fat

- helps move cholesterol out of our bloodstream, protecting our heart

- helps keep our bowels moving regularly by absorbing and bulking up faeces into nice soft stools

- feeds the good bugs in our intestines, keeping our gut microbiome happy. (More about the microbiome in Chapter 7.)

Which fibre is best?

Fibre is a form of carbs, made up of the indigestible parts of plants. It's in fruit and vegetables (particularly leafy green vegetables and pulses), whole oats and other whole grains. There are a number of different types of fibre, and research is ongoing into their different effects.

---

[34] According to the latest Australian National Nutrition and Physical Activity Survey, less than 20% of Australian adults meet the suggested dietary target of 28–38 g of fibre per day.

The central message is that we should consume more fibre from *non-starchy vegetables, fruit, pulses, whole oats and barley*. And to reach and maintain a healthy weight, *include psyllium fibre* every day as well.

Psyllium husk is the powdery husk of seeds from the *Plantago ovata* plant. Buy plain psyllium husk at any health food shop or supermarket. Don't bother with psyllium capsules: they have only 1–2 g fibre per serve, and that's not going to get you even close to where you need to be. At nearly 10 times the price of plain loose psyllium, they're also ridiculously expensive.

Avoid manufactured or synthetic fibre supplements. Processed fibre is generally artificially produced cellulose, and often flavoured and coloured. Many forms also contain inulin, a substance that's generally healthy, but contributes to digestive upset in people who are sensitive to fermenting carbs (FODMAPs). Processed fibre supplements are less effective for maintaining healthy weight (and relieving constipation), than psyllium.

The daily dose

Put one tablespoon of psyllium into a large, dry glass, and fill with water while stirring constantly. If you're not used to fibre, start with a teaspoon per day and increase gradually.

Allow it to sit for 20 seconds and give it another stir, as it will have separated a bit. Then gulp it down in one go. This is not something to savour. Fill the glass once more, stirring to pick up the bits stuck to the edges, and drink that too.

All done until tomorrow.

HABIT HELPERS – THE RIGHT CARBS

Get your priorities straight. Non-starchy vegetables first, including lots of greens, then unprocessed protein and fat. Carbs last.

Know your zones. When out shopping, make a quick mental assessment of food you see. Is it green, amber or red zone? Danger zone? Notice, too, where different foods are displayed in a supermarket. Red zone and danger carbs are likely to be in premium positions: eye-level shelves, aisle ends, and at the checkout.

Not so fast! Avoid fast food, and limit most takeaway and restaurant food. Even in 'high end' restaurants (and even in savoury food), cooking methods frequently include a lot of sugar and other carbs. Chapter 10 has more about navigating restaurants and cafes.

Nice and natural. Get your carbs from unprocessed sources, as close to nature as you can.

Go low after lunch. Don't have starchy vegetables, grains or pasta for dinner. Studies suggest that, especially for individuals who are less tolerant of carbs, carbs eaten later in the day are more likely to end up stored as fat (Chapter 3 has more on meal timing).

REFLECTIONS

- How much fibre are you getting? Make a rough estimate based on a typical day (use the online Australian Food Composition Database to work it out).

The wrong carbs – filler foods

Filler foods – sugar and the danger zone

Filler foods – sugar and danger zone food – play a special role in overeating, overweight and obesity, which is why they deserve their own chapter. They're a big part of what's making us fat. Eating these things *will prevent us* from reaching a healthy weight.

Quitting filler food is the single most effective thing you can do to regain your happy weight, and good health.

Sugar occurs naturally in fruit, sweeter vegetables, honey and milk. Having a little sugar in its natural form now and then is fine. The problems arise when concentrated forms of sugar (whether natural or refined) become part of our everyday eating. And unfortunately there's a lot of sugar around.

The danger zone happens when red zone carbs – refined sugar and refined grains, mostly in the form of white flour – meet fat and extra sugar or salt, or sugary or salty flavours.

Weight gain

Filler foods cause us to gain excess weight. They're high in sugar, refined carbs and unhealthy fats, and often include other ingredients that aren't classified as food. The carb content is metabolised quickly into glucose, and from there, it's mostly stored as fat.

Empty calories

Filler foods provide little or no protein, fibre, vitamins or minerals. They just fill us up, taking up space for no return. They leave no room in our tummy or time in our day, or perhaps money in our wallet, to buy, prepare and eat the things that nurture and nourish our bodies: eating filler foods means missing out on nutrients.

... And addictive

Filler foods, particularly danger zone foods, fuel overeating: we keep craving them. The combination of high sugar or starch, and high fat, makes our brain release the feel-good hormone dopamine. To get another hit, we seek out these foods again and again.

The food manufacturing industry calls filler food 'discretionary food'. They imply that it's entirely our choice to eat it. And that by extension, if we eat too much, it's our own greed or lack of willpower that will see us put on weight.

Neither of these things is true. Research shows filler foods have high addictive potential, and it's no accident.

Recognising filler food

Filler foods don't occur in nature. They're processed products, usually offered in bright, attractive packaging. They're often also cheap. Supermarkets frequently discount them to bring us into the supermarket, or encourage us to make an impulse buy.

Sugar

Sugar – is it as bad as they say? In a word – *yes*. If you aren't ready to stop it altogether, then reduce as much as you can, especially added sugar.

The more sugar you can eliminate, the easier it will be to reach your ideal weight, and stay there. Sugar adds nothing; it's just a mirage.

Apart from its addictive quality, there are other sinister things about sugar. A diet high in sugar changes our gut microbiome – the happy community of millions of different bugs that live mainly in our intestines. The changes aren't good; they disrupt the way our gut communicates with our brain, and encourage over-growth of the wrong types of bacteria. Chapter 7 has more about the gut microbiome.

Added sugar

We add sugar when we put it in tea or coffee, spread it on toast or add it to cooking. But it's also lurking in many processed foods and drinks (savoury as well as sweet). And not just junk food, either – many foods that claim to be a healthier choice have significant amounts of added sugar. Muesli bars, breakfast drinks or bars, flavoured yoghurt and dried fruit and nut snack mixes, are all examples of high-sugar foods marketed as 'good for you'.

Other unexpected sources of added sugar include:

- *Savoury processed food* such as flavoured potato chips, flavoured canned tuna, canned or powdered soup.

- *Sauces* such as soy sauce, BBQ sauce, tomato sauce and mayonnaise, and most restaurant and cafe sauces and dressings, including on the nice green-vegetable salad you just ordered.

- *Prepared cooking ingredients* such as spaghetti sauces or 'cook in the pan' sauces to add to meat or vegetable dishes.

- *Restaurant- and cafe-made savoury dishes* including soups, stir-fries, curries and noodle dishes.

- *Fast food* such as pizza, burgers and BBQ chicken.

Sugar by any other name…

Sugar is usually added in the form of cane sugar, but it can also be from other sources, like corn or maple syrup, or fruit juice concentrate. It's all sugar, and it all takes us further from our ideal weight.

Food labels describe sugar in all sorts of ways, including:

- glucose, sucrose or fructose
- dextrose and maltose
- brown sugar and molasses
- icing sugar
- fruit sugar syrup, fruit juice concentrate and cane juice
- malt powder
- rapadura (the first pressing of the sugar cane, dried to make granules)
- agave syrup, maple syrup, rice bran syrup and honey.

Food manufacturers may hide added sugar in 'healthy' food by using honey, sweet fruit or fruit juice. Grape juice is frequently added to canned fruit, and fruit juice concentrate sweetens up any number of products. Dates are used as the base ingredient for that protein ball. Agave nectar in the vegan choc-mint slice.

How much added sugar?

Aim for as little added sugar as possible. At most – six teaspoons (24 g) per day for women, nine teaspoons (36 g) for men. ***Never have more than 10 g at any meal or snack.***

Find the sugar content of packaged food by reading the nutrition panel and ingredients list:

> ***Nutrition panel:*** find 'total carbohydrates', then 'sugar'. If sugar is more than *15 g per 100 g, or more than 10 g per serve, it's too high.*

> ***Ingredients list:*** Sugar must be shown in the ingredients, but it might go by other names (e.g. fruit juice concentrate or syrup). Look out for some sneaky labelling, which may scatter different sugars through the ingredient list. If sugar by any name is in the top three, the product is likely to be too high in sugar. You can make an exception for products used in small quantities, like chilli sauce.

Sugar-free sweeteners

There are many non-sugar sweeteners available, with varying benefits and downsides compared with plain sugar.[35] Avoid all of them; they're likely to be making us fatter.

Although non-sugar sweeteners do not raise blood sugar, some observational studies link regular consumption to weight gain,

---

[35] The sugar-free sweeteners are: *Artificial sweeteners*, including aspartame (including NutraSweet™ and Equal®) (951), saccharin (954), acesulfame K and sucralose (Splenda®); *Sugar alcohols* such as sorbitol, maltitol, xylitol and erythritol; and *Plant-derived sweeteners*, mainly stevia and monk fruit.

obesity and risk of type 2 diabetes and metabolic syndrome. Clinical trials vary in their findings, and it is likely that different types of sweeteners behave differently in our bodies. While there is still controversy over whether non-sugar sweeteners contribute to weight gain, there is at least no good evidence that they help with weight reduction.

There are a few theories about why non-sugar sweeteners might be linked to weight gain.

One theory is that eating sweet-tasting things leads us to seek out more sweet-tasting things, increasing the likelihood that we will overeat. Even if they contain no sugar, sweet things release dopamine into our brain. We have evolved to seek out dopamine, and our bodies have learned that sweet food is an excellent dopamine trigger, so that's what we go for. Whether it's sweetened naturally or artificially, we're still feeding the desire and encouraging over-eating.

Some studies suggest that when we eat non-sugar sweeteners, the brain notices the difference and feels 'tricked', so it seeks out even more carbs. A related idea is that when we have non-sugar sweetened food we subconsciously register this food as not 'counting' in our energy intake, and overeat other foods.

Another theory is that things that taste sweet (even when there is no sugar) make our body release insulin, triggering the process that ensures any energy that we don't need right away will be stored as fat. And another theory is that regularly using non-sugar sweeteners disrupts our gut microbiome in a way that leads to weight gain.

Whatever the reason, *eating sweet-tasting substances is likely to feed sugar cravings and sugar dependence*. My advice is to steer clear of sweeteners, whether natural or artificial.

Fructose – what's it all about?

Fructose is the sugar found naturally in fruit, and it also makes up 50% of ordinary cane sugar (the other half is glucose). Fructose can also be manufactured by processing sugar cane, sugar beet or corn, and used as an intense sweetener. Concentrated fruit juice is also widely used as a sweetener. It's difficult to avoid fructose if you eat anything sweet.

There are metabolic reasons to be cautious about fructose. While some is processed in our gut, any 'overflow' needs to be broken down primarily by the liver. When our liver deals with fructose it produces triglycerides, which are a type of fat. Triglycerides produced from fructose are more likely to be stored as visceral fat, which dangerously collects around our internal organs. Much of the fat created by excess fructose remains in the liver, contributing to development of non-alcoholic fatty liver disease. High fructose intake is also associated with insulin resistance, which is a precursor to type 2 diabetes. And to top it off, the process of metabolising fructose also produces free radicals, which damage cells.

There is ongoing research into fructose and its role in fatty liver, obesity and diabetes. Until we know more – the best bet is to *go natural*:

- Limit fructose in your diet to what you get from *whole fruit only*, and say no to fruit juice.
- Read food labels and avoid fructose and concentrated fruit sugars.
- *Limit sugar intake overall.*

The danger zone

Think of the foods that have you reaching for more – and more. Potato chips? Soy chips? Pizza? Cake? Donuts? Chocolate biscuits?

They all have something in common – they're made with *starch, a big dose of fat, and extra sugar and/or salt.*

This potently flavoursome combination actively hinders our attempts to reach or keep our best weight. Danger zone foods override our sense of fullness – and our sense of judgement. The formula is highly attractive, to the point of addiction. A number of studies and reviews have concluded that the way our brain reacts to food made from processed carbs with fat and flavouring is very different from its reaction to other types of food, and is associated with symptoms of addiction.

It's very easy to overeat danger zone foods, and they cause cravings for more. Processed food manufacturers use the formula because it keeps us coming back.

Recognising the danger zone

Danger zone food is carb-based: usually refined, red zone starches, but sometimes amber or even green zone carbs are prepared in the danger zone. Danger zone food made from otherwise high-quality carbs includes deep-fried puffed chickpeas, salted lentil crisps, and veggie chips.

The common thread is the mix of starch, fat and flavouring. *Be aware, and avoid it.*

Nature does not make food in the danger zone. You can find starches with a little fat, but only a tiny amount of sugar (for example a grain of wheat). You can also find starches with high natural sugars, but they contain only trace amounts of fat (for example sweet corn and bananas).

Danger zone examples

The sweet	*The salty*	*The sweet and salty*
Donuts	Hot potato chips	Chocolate-covered pretzel
Waffles and churros	Potato crisps	Salted chocolate
Sweet biscuits, pastries	Salted buttered popcorn	Salted caramel anything: popcorn, potato crisps, ice cream…
Cakes and most desserts		

What about 'treat food'?

Food presented to us as a 'treat' is frequently danger zone food. Take a step back to work out why we've been conditioned to see something that is not good for us in any way, as a treat. Is it because of powerful advertising? Or because we have it at special times, so it's tightly tied to good feelings? Or because it's a hyper-flavoursome thing, which studies suggest may be physiologically addictive? Push back, and let your self-care override the conditioning.

Of course this doesn't mean 'never again'. Once at your target weight, you'll be able to eat occasional danger zone food without it leading to weight gain. But you also might decide that what you once saw as a treat isn't worth it, especially if it's something that you find addictive or triggering.

If you do eat danger zone food, then:

Keep it (really) small. A very small amount will not cause blood glucose to rise too high or too quickly, and there will be less excess energy to be stored as fat.

Make it rare. We're talking perhaps monthly. Maybe weekly. Certainly not daily, or multiple times per week.

Do it consciously. Be mindful of the addictive potential of the starch/fat/flavouring combination that makes up most of what we have been conditioned to think of as treats.

Don't buy the advertising. Advertisers are determined, and not to be underestimated. They present us with danger zone foods at every opportunity, trying to convince us that they are 'treats' that we 'deserve'. Don't let them suck you in. *Your body does not deserve to be treated badly.*

Clean out your cupboards

I know this is a typical 'start the diet' piece of advice, but there's good reason for it. Be truthful to yourself about what's in your cupboards.

The most important things to find and remove are the danger zone items. Chuck out the chips, cake, biscuits, chocolate and lollies. In the compost or council organic waste bin. Don't give it away, it's not going to help anyone.

After you've cleaned out any danger zone stuff, it's time to get more specific. Read the labels of anything left in the pantry, fridge or freezer that's in a packet:

- If it has more than 10 g of sugar per serve, *or* more than 15 g of sugar per 100 g (or 100 ml), get rid of it.

- If it's over the 'sugar limit' but it's something you use only in small amounts and not often (such as cooking sauces and marinades) keep it, but remember the sugar content when you use it.

HABIT HELPERS – LIMITING FILLER FOODS

Shake off the sugar. The more you remove filler foods from your diet, the easier it will be to reach your ideal weight, and stay there.

Be aware. Understand why you might crave filler foods. Make your own conscious choice about whether you'll eat it, why and how much.

Steer clear of sweeteners and stop feeding sugar dependence. Non-sugar sweeteners are commonly used in low-calorie foods marketed as 'better for you', such as flavoured yoghurts, milks and kombucha.

Love the labels. To limit sugar in your supermarket shopping, get used to reading the labels of packaged foods. Reject products with more 10 g of sugar per serve, or more than 15 g per 100 g. Stay away from highly processed foods. (Test it – if you had the time and skill, could you make this at home, with ordinary ingredients?)

Truth in the trolley. If you don't buy sugar or danger zone food, you won't have it in the house (or by your desk). So – never shop on an empty tummy, or if you might be triggered by worry, stress or sadness.

> ***Cravings?*** Filler foods tend to be addictive, so you may experience withdrawal and cravings. Chapter 10 has ideas for breaking free from filler-food cravings.
>
> ***Get picky.*** Think it. Say it. *'That type of food's not good enough for me'. 'I don't eat sugar'.* Keep your commitment front of mind.
>
> ***Defer it.*** *'Not right now, thanks; maybe I'll have some later'.* (Maybe you will. Or maybe not.)

REFLECTIONS

Carbs and the danger zone

- What types of sugar are in your daily diet? What are the sources of that sugar?

- Have a look at some of your fridge and pantry 'staples' – the things you eat at least once a week. Check the labels:

  » Is sugar in the top three ingredients?

  » What is the total carb content per 100 g? And the separately listed 'sugar' content?

  » What are the other ingredients? Is there any vegetable oil, or ingredients you don't recognise?

- What red zone carbs do you eat; how often and how much? What about danger zone food?

- Identify triggers for buying filler food. And what triggers you to eat it. Go deeper than just 'I like it' – *why* do you like it? Is it the texture, the look, the smell, the flavour? An association with a happy event or time? Or to fit in with other people?

- What will help you change the way you think and feel about these products? What will help you stay in charge of whether you eat them or not?

Recap – What to eat

What's the problem? Most of us aren't eating enough vegetables and fibre, and are eating too much unhelpful stuff (mostly the wrong sort of carbs).

What to do about it?

- *Eat more vegetables*, especially greens and other non-starchy vegetables.

- *Eat more fibre.* It's not just for keeping our bowels moving. Use psyllium as a supplement.

- *Eat plenty of good-quality protein.*

- *Eat enough good-quality fat* from mostly unprocessed plants sources (nuts, seeds and cold-pressed oils) and fish.

CHAPTER FIVE

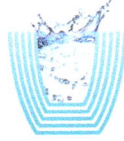

WHAT TO DRINK

What to drink? More water.

Water is essential for life. No doubt you're drinking enough for life, but chances are you aren't drinking enough for your best health. Drinking more water can help you reach and maintain your ideal weight.

In this chapter, we'll look at:

- why it's important to **drink more water**, aiming for at least three litres per day – and working out a routine to make sure you get it

- how drinking water can help *manage appetite and portion sizes*

- *what not to drink*, and the role of alcohol.

Drink more water

Most Australians don't drink nearly enough water.

Statistics from the most recent survey of national nutrition and physical activity showed only 22% of us meet daily recommendations for fluid intake. Individual water needs vary depending on our environment, activity levels and metabolism, but according to the Australian National Health and Medical Research Council, we should drink on average 2.1–2.6 litres per day on top of the fluids we get from food. More in hot climates or if we're very active.[36]

But for reasons we'll look at in this section, we should be aiming at water intake that is better-than-adequate, because it helps reduce and manage weight. While there's variation between individuals, I recommend close to *three litres per day* on top of moisture in food. More if you're exercising a lot, or outside during hot weather.

Be guided by urine colour – if it's a very pale yellow, you're probably having enough.

Important to know – medical conditions

If you have *congestive heart failure or impaired kidney function*, fluid intake needs to be carefully regulated, and your doctor will have talked to you about this. People with liver failure or protein deficiency, or taking steroids, are also at risk of over-hydration.

If this is you: *don't* drink more water.

---

[36] The NHMRC guide is based on an estimated average turnover of water of 4% of our total body weight each day, and the observed impacts of dehydration by as little as 2% of our body weight. The origin of the 4% is shrouded in mystery, but it possibly dates from a 1920s study of kidney excretion in the United Kingdom. A more recent US study on water metabolism (2003) concluded that the average range of usual total water intake from food and drink is 3 litres in men, and 2.5 in women.

Water helps reduce weight

Many clinical studies have observed that drinking more water helps to reduce excess body fat. For example, a number of randomised controlled trials have found that participants who 'preloaded' with water (between 500 ml and 1 litre) before each main meal had *significantly* lower BMI and body fat than the control group over trial periods of 8 to 12 weeks. One of these studies also tracked fasting blood sugar, triglycerides (fats circulating in the bloodstream) and LDL cholesterol, finding that these measurements, as well as BMI and waist circumference, were lower in the water-drinking group.[37]

Complementing the clinical studies are studies of large groups of people over time, showing that those with higher total water intake (counting both food and drink) generally have lower body fat and waist circumference, and that drinking more plain water is associated with lower risks of weight gain. Underhydration is significantly associated with obesity, high waist circumference and metabolic syndrome.[38]

There are varying theories about why water has such an effect, and it's *probably a combination of reasons*, including the following:

Reduces the amount we eat during a meal. Studies show that for most people, drinking a couple of glasses of water about 30 minutes before a meal naturally suppresses appetite and reduces the energy consumed at that meal.

Replaces calorific drinks. Drinking water instead of a sweetened drink, milk or juice, materially cuts our overall sugar and calorie intake.

---

[37] Sedaghat (2021) Effect of pre-meal water intake on the serum levels of copeptin, glycemic control, lipid profile and anthropometric indices in patients with type 2 diabetes mellitus: a randomized, controlled trial.

[38] E.g. Stookey (2020) Underhydration is associated with obesity, chronic diseases, and death within 3 to 6 years in the U.S. population aged 51-70 years; Walton (2019) Cross-sectional association of dietary water intakes and sources, and adiposity: National Adult Nutrition Survey, the Republic of Ireland; Pan (2020) Plain water intake and association with the risk of overweight in the Chinese adult population: China Health and Nutrition Survey 2006-2011.

May increase metabolism. Some studies have shown that drinking water speeds up our metabolism, increasing the amount of 'resting energy' we use, whereas others showed no such effect. In the studies that did show an effect, it was significant, with 500 ml (two large glasses) of water increasing resting metabolism by 10–30% for about an hour. Some studies have also shown that drinking cold water uses even more energy, partly because our body needs to work harder to bring it up to body temperature.

Helps digestive system function. Drinking water helps break down food, and helps move food down into our stomach. It also helps keep things soft and moving steadily through our intestines, so drinking plenty of water helps combat constipation.

Increases fat burning. This is one I like a lot. Drinking plenty of water leads to greater fat burning and lower blood sugar. The most likely reason seems to be that *cells increase their volume when we drink water* (but not other fluids). And plump, well-hydrated cells promote fat oxidation (that is, use of fat stores for energy). Dehydrated cells on the other hand are less able to metabolise fat. This may have a further downside for healthy weight – a chronically dehydrated person's body is less able to use fat stores and is therefore looking constantly for glucose (from carbs) as its main source of energy.

How much is too much?

It *is* possible to drink too much water – and that can be fatal. Too much water can result in loss of electrolytes from your bloodstream; in particular, sodium. Dangerously low levels of sodium cause excessive swelling, which in brain cells can be fatal.

It's rare to drink enough to cause such a dramatic dilution in sodium levels, but it can happen. People at most risk are those with kidney disease, heart or liver failure or protein deficiency, or taking steroids or intravenous fluids. Athletes or others doing hard physical labour who are sweating out electrolytes without replacing them may also be at risk.

People with normal kidney function can handle up to 800 ml per hour. The three litres per day I'm recommending is well below this. *Just don't drink it all at once.*

When to drink

Drink regularly

Many of us only drink if reminded to, or as a habit if we're used to drinking at mealtimes. Sometimes we may not even drink when we're thirsty, or we might eat instead.

This weak signalling of a need to drink shouldn't be surprising – our first food as infants (milk) is nearly 90% water. And the line between what is food and drink is quite blurred, as many high-calorie foods are presented as drinks or semi-liquids – soft drinks, soups, energy drinks and protein shakes. And both eating and drinking provide sensory 'reward' – we have the sensation of something in our mouth, tongue, taste buds, throat and stomach.

So don't rely on 'feeling thirsty' – just drink regularly. Urine should be a pale straw colour.

Drink even if you aren't thirsty

Some research suggests that people who are overweight, and people who don't drink enough water, do not feel thirsty – a vicious circle, which results in drinking even less. Studies show that being chronically under-hydrated leads to chronic cell shrinkage, a condition that can discourage your body from burning its fat stores. The antidote is to drink more, whether you feel thirsty or not. Your body is likely to re-learn the thirst signal.

Drink when you feel a need to put something in your mouth

When you're not sure what you want to put in your mouth – drink water. Another way to put it: if the 'wanting' something to put in your mouth is in your head (an idea) rather than a gnawing in your stomach (hunger) – drink instead.

Drink to reduce appetite

Water physically takes up room in our stomach, helping to reduce the amount we eat at the next meal. Take advantage of this by drinking a couple of glasses (about 500 ml) 20–30 minutes before each meal.

Get into a routine

Each time you drink, have 1.5–2 large glasses. When I say 'large glass', I mean 250 ml. Find a glass that's 250 ml and hang on to it.

Work out a routine that fits into your daily life, as adopting this new habit will take a bit of forethought and planning. My suggestions are:

- On rising – have a tablespoon of psyllium with two large glasses of water.

- Fill water bottles or jugs with about two litres of water. Keep them on the kitchen bench or desk, where you see them all the time. Drink steadily through the day. If you're going to be out and about, fill and carry a one-litre bottle and empty it twice during the day.

- Drink two large glasses 20–30 minutes before each meal.

- Aim to finish 2.5 litres before 5 pm.

- During the day, have at least one large pot of herbal tea (or two large cups, if you don't have a pot). I recommend you acquire a nice teapot. There's something special and comforting about tea from a pot.

- As soon as you get home – have two large glasses of water.

Drinking a lot of water means needing the toilet a lot too. Plan ahead, and go when you have the opportunity. If you miss the toilet stop, use the opportunity to strengthen your bladder and pelvic floor. But don't overdo it – excessively hanging on for long periods can put you at risk of urinary tract infections.

Aim **not to drink much after 7 pm**, or you'll be up for the loo disturbing your sleep, and good sleep is essential to happy weight.

Eating while drinking?

There's a bit of debate about whether to avoid drinking and eating at the same time.

The 'don't drink while you eat' camp says that water dilutes the enzymes and acids that our stomach and saliva make to help digest food. However, there is no evidence to support this, and it is more likely that the stomach and mouth respond immediately as they are physiologically designed to, by making more enzymes and acids.

Personally, too much water with a meal makes me feel bloated and uncomfortable, and I'd rather my stomach not be stretched in that way, or forced into acid-producing overdrive. My recommendation is to hydrate before meals, and at other times during the day.

HABIT HELPERS – DRINK MORE WATER

Have it cold. Drink water cold if you can. Cold water forces our body to use energy to bring the water to body temperature.

Carry it around. Keep your water bottle close by, where you see it frequently.

Twice as nice. When you reach for your water – drink two glasses or half a bottle (400 ml).

Add some interest. If you're not keen on plain water, try infusing it with herbs (fresh mint or basil, cinnamon or fennel seeds) or pieces of fruit – orange, lime or a few berries. It will infuse faster at room temperature.

> *Water while you wait*. Each time you're in a waiting pattern –
> e.g. waiting for your computer to boot up, the kettle to boil,
> or your turn in the bathroom – have a glass of water.
>
> *Delaying tactics*. If you're thinking about food and it's not a
> mealtime, have two glasses of water and wait half an hour. If
> you're properly hungry, you will know when the half hour is
> up, and the water 'preload' will help you eat a smaller portion.
>
> *Take it easy*. Don't drink more than 800 ml per hour (unless
> you're doing heavy physical activity in a hot or dry climate,
> and replace electrolytes regularly).

REFLECTIONS

- How much water do you normally drink, and what will
  you do to get to 3 litres a day?

- Since you started reading, have you increased your intake?
  How did you do this? If it was difficult, what will you do
  to make sure the habit sticks?

What to drink

We need plain water, not extra calories or other substances, so just
drink more water. Always have water in preference to fruit juice,
milk or sugar-sweetened drinks.

What not to drink

Soft drinks aren't the only type of sweetened drink to watch out
for – flavoured milk is also high in sugar, as is fruit juice, even if it
has 'no added sugar'.

Avoid:

- fruit juice and sweetened milk
- soft drinks, including iced tea
- vitamin waters, energy drinks and sports drinks
- drinks sweetened with non-sugar sweeteners.

Cut down on:

- caffeine in tea, coffee and energy drinks
- alcohol.

Carbs in drinks – milk, juice and sugar

Milk, juice and sweetened drinks all have carbs in the form of natural or added sugars (or both). They raise blood sugar significantly and quickly, and if you don't use that fuel straight away, it will get stored as fat.

Although plain milk has good nutritional value (protein, fat and calcium), it's still a significant source of carbs and raises blood sugar quickly, whether skim or full fat. Flavoured milk falls into the same category as fruit juice and other sweetened drinks.

Fruit juice, even juice without added sugar, is still *high in sugar*. Although it contains vitamins (mostly vitamin C), these are also found in high quantities in plenty of other foods – and in whole fruit too, of course.

Caffeine

We're sometimes told that caffeine is a diuretic, and that it removes more water from our body than it supplies. In very large quantities this might be so, but there is no evidence that moderate consumption (around four cups per day) has a dehydrating effect.

Caffeine has other side effects, though – it can increase our levels of cortisol (a stress hormone), and interfere with our circadian rhythm and sleep. Chronically high cortisol and poor sleep both contribute to weight gain; more about this in Chapter 8.

If you're sensitive to caffeine, keep it under three cups per day, and avoid it in the afternoon.

Add milk if you like, as it's a good source of calcium. Just be aware that your small flat white contains around 150 ml of milk, minimum. That's about 8 g of carbs. Leave out the sugar and artificial sweeteners.

Tea

Black tea, green tea and white tea are all made from the leaves of the camellia plant. Drying and fermenting the leaves, and different varieties of the plant, give tea varying flavours and colours.

'Herbal tea', on the other hand, is a tisane or infusion of plants, flowers and other substances. It usually doesn't contain caffeine.

Black, green and white tea are high in caffeine and other stimulating substances. Herbal tisanes containing yerba mate, ginseng and guarana are also stimulating, and not good for bedtime.

Green tea? Yes please!

Green tea is not only a good source of water, it also has other significant health benefits, including as an antioxidant, and an aid to weight management.

Green tea has a thermogenic effect, so it raises our metabolism. It's also associated with decreased fasting blood sugar and promotes fat burning (oxidation), although the precise mechanism for this is not known.

Green tea is high in tannin and can make you feel nauseous on an empty stomach, so have it with or after food.

Different types of water

Tap water or sparkling, filtered, mineral, soda, alkaline, spring... There's no difference in terms of hydration, and in most of Australia we have excellent quality drinking water, straight from the tap.

Looking for bottled water? Be aware that it's crazily expensive. Tap water, on the other hand, costs a fraction of one cent per litre if you're paying the water bill (or nothing if you're not). Most Australian bottled water is simply bore water, pumped up from underground, and must have one of the highest profit margins of all packaged foods.

And while we're on packaging – the bottles are a major problem. The energy used to produce plastic bottles is considerable, and only about one in five plastic bottles gets recycled – the rest end up buried in landfill, or worse, in the litter stream, where they'll most likely find their way to the ocean. Plastic, including microplastic once the bottle degrades into tiny pieces, is the number one threat to marine ecosystems.

Worried about sodium in soda, sparkling or spring water?

Sparkling and spring water are sometimes thought of as high in sodium, but they normally aren't. Levels vary a lot between different brands, but most are well under 10 mg sodium per litre. Check the label if you're concerned, and aim for less than 20 mg per litre.

Sodium in tap water varies considerably across Australia; although it's mostly quite low, it can be up to 300 mg per litre or more. For most people this isn't a problem, but if you're on a low-sodium diet, it's a good idea to check with your water provider.

Alkaline water

Alkaline water is water that contains alkaline minerals to lower the acidity (pH) of the water. It also has 'negative oxidation reduction potential', which means it will have an antioxidant effect. The claim is that drinking an alkaline substance can neutralise acidity in your body, which, in turn, will keep your body healthy.

So… if antioxidants are good, and neutralising acid in your body is good too – isn't alkaline water going to be very good for you, even better than plain water?

The short answer is that there isn't good evidence to support the theory, although that won't stop food manufacturers from wanting to sell us alkaline water. Our body is excellent at regulating its own acidity within a very narrow range – and we'd die if it didn't do this. Luckily for us, dietary changes don't alter the pH of our blood or any other part of our body (except momentarily, while the body returns to its natural pH levels).

If you drink alkaline water, check the label to ensure it contains minerals that should be present in your water, including magnesium and calcium. Alkaline water that's been produced by reverse osmosis won't contain these minerals unless they've been added.

You can make your own if you want to – add ¼ teaspoon of bicarbonate (baking soda) to a large glass of water to increase its alkalinity. That's it.

Sugar-added water – soft drink by another name

Soft drink manufacturers are very aware that consumers are onto them in terms of health, and will do everything they can to have us continue to buy things in bottles from them.

New drinks are coming onto the market every year advertised as 'healthy' because they aren't soft drinks as we're used to seeing them. There's only one thing you really need to look for – sugar content. If the drink contains sugar, it isn't going to give the health benefits of plain water. Just extra calories on your daily intake.

'Vitamin water' is a relatively new entrant to the soft drink market. There are now a range of brands of these flavoured drinks with added vitamins – usually at least vitamin C and some of the B-group vitamins. They're marketed as healthy, and have elegant, healthy-sounding names. But they contain added sugar (including often pure fructose), non-sugar sweeteners or sometimes both. Get your vitamins and minerals from vegetables and fruit, and your water from plain water.

Coconut water

Coconut water is the clear fluid inside not-quite-ripe coconuts. It contains natural electrolytes – manganese, potassium and sodium, in varying amounts depending on ripeness of the coconut. So far, so good.

Coconut water straight from a coconut also contains significant amounts of sugar – 6.6 g per 100 ml, which is more than three teaspoons per glass. Packaged coconut water generally also contains added sugar. Treat it with caution, and drink water instead.

Vinegar

Do have a daily dose of up to 30 ml (1 tablespoon) of good-quality, unfiltered, unpasteurised, aged vinegar, diluted in water.

A number of human and animal studies over the last decade have demonstrated significant beneficial effects of vinegar. Among other things, vinegar seems to help maintain stable blood sugar, improve metabolism of carbs, reduce the size of fat cells, and increase the use of body fat as energy. Unfiltered, unpasteurised vinegar is also a probiotic that improves the diversity of good bugs in our gut microbiome.

Use a good-quality vinegar such as *unfiltered, unpasteurised apple cider vinegar or an aged rice vinegar such as Chinese Shanxi aged vinegar or Japanese Kurosu*. Different types of vinegar have slightly different properties and other potential health benefits, but the acetic acid in all of them is the main reason why vinegar is a useful aid in weight reduction.

Drink vinegar in water just before, or during, a meal. Use it in dressings for salads and vegetables.

Diluted, with a straw!

Vinegar is extremely acidic, and (even when diluted) will strip the enamel from your teeth. Drinking neat vinegar is a serious assault on the delicate skin of your throat and oesophagus, and can cause burns and ulcers.

Dilute vinegar in water and drink it through a straw. Rinse your mouth with plain water afterwards.

Juicing – healthy or not?

I'm not a fan of juicing. Even vegetable-only juicing, which is mostly fine in terms of sugar content, fills you up with… well, juice. Yes, nutrients too, but minus effective fibre, and without the physical act of chewing. *If your goal is weight reduction – juicing isn't helpful.*

If you really feel like you need the intense micronutrient boost you'll get from vegetable juicing, do it. But make up the fibre elsewhere in your diet, and don't let it replace good chewing habits. Chapter 4 has more on juicing.

Alcohol

Take care with alcohol. There's more detail about it in the next section.

HABIT HELPERS – WHAT TO DRINK

Choose water above other things. Infuse it with lemon slices or mint sprigs for variety.

Notice the competition. Notice how sweetened drinks (including those using non-sugar sweeteners) are all around us, and they're heavily advertised. It's intentional. Avoid or limit them.

Beware the booze. There are many reasons to be wary of alcohol, including the significant risk of cancer.

REFLECTIONS

Fruit juice and soft drinks

- Do you drink soft drinks? How often, and are they sugar- or non-sugar sweetened? How will you reduce or stop drinking these?

- What about fruit juice or flavoured milk?

Caffeine

- What's your caffeine intake like? If you're having it with sugar or sweeteners, when and how will you cut it out?

- What caffeine-free alternatives do you enjoy, or will you try?

Alcohol

For many people, me included, alcohol is a part of life. It's part of many formal and informal occasions, both happy and sad. But it's important to *significantly limit* the amount we drink.

This isn't a book about the dangers of alcohol, nor is it an attempt to stop anyone from drinking. But it's important to acknowledge that alcohol has impacts on healthy eating. Too much alcohol, especially alcohol with extra sugar (e.g. alcopops, beer, white and sparkling wine, spirits with soft drink mixers), undermines healthy eating habits and will get in the way of your efforts to reduce weight.

If you feel that you aren't in control of your drinking, seek out expert advice and help. Take it seriously; it's too easy to brush it off or rationalise it.

Alcohol = empty calories

Alcohol is not food. It has **no nutritional value**, and contains nothing that our bodies need. Even so, alcohol does still contain calories. Gram for gram, pure alcohol has more calories than sugar, and only a little less than fat.[39]

In terms of (un)healthy eating, alcohol is up there with refined sugars.

Most alcoholic drinks also contain some carbs – the amount depends on the type of drink. Beer, sweet liquors, alcopops and spirits with mixers are highest in carbs.

The total calories do add up:

- one 150 ml glass of dry red or white wine (average restaurant serve) – about 120 calories
- one double-shot (60 ml) glass of spirits (no mixer) – about 120 calories
- one 375 ml can of 5% alcohol beer – about 140 calories
- one 275 ml bottle of vodka pre-mix – at least 150 calories, depending on the flavour.

For comparison, one chocolate-coated, cream-filled chocolate biscuit has about 100 calories.

Alcohol, particularly alcohol in the evenings, is a common cause of excess calories too close to bedtime.

Alcohol is metabolised ahead of anything else

When we drink alcohol, our body immediately diverts its attention to metabolising it. This means it's using only alcohol for fuel, preventing us from burning any other source of fuel, including fat or carbs, until it's dealt with the alcohol.

---

[39] One gram of alcohol yields seven calories, while a gram of protein or carb yields four calories. One gram of fat is nine calories.

Alcohol can lead to overeating

Apart from being 'empty calories', drinking alcohol before or with a meal dulls our normal sense that we've had enough to eat. In other words, alcohol can easily lead to overeating. Drinks and nibbles with friends, bar snacks…

Alcohol increases cortisol

Although alcohol might make us feel relaxed, in fact it increases our levels of cortisol, the stress hormone. Chronically increased cortisol leads us to eat more of the wrong food, and to tend to store excess fat in our abdomen – a particularly dangerous place for it to be. Chapter 8 has more about cortisol.

Alcohol is a diuretic

Alcohol is dehydrating because it reduces the production of one of the hormones that regulates our water levels, and as a result, we urinate more than the volume of water contained in the alcoholic drink. And we can't totally offset this effect by simply drinking more water. This is one cause of the hangover headache, and a big contributor to wrinkled, saggy skin.

Alcohol is a health risk – including for cancer

Alcohol is never completely safe. There is no level at which we can be sure that alcohol is not harming our health, and no level at which it improves health.

When we drink, our body metabolises alcohol into a chemical called acetaldehyde. Acetaldehyde is a likely carcinogen, and presumed to be a key reason why alcohol increases our risks of a number of cancers, especially breast cancer. Alcohol is also linked to high blood pressure, heart disease, stroke and injury.

Despite these undisputed facts, residents in most of the so-called 'Blue Zones', where people live unusually long and healthy lives, do drink wine.[40] They generally drink daily, with family or friends and with a meal, *but only in small quantities*. Alcohol intake in these communities is also combined with many other important lifestyle elements, including lower calorie, plant-based diets that are *naturally low in refined carbs*. It's far more likely that their good health is due to the absence of processed foods, rather than the presence of alcohol.

Support weight goals by reducing alcohol

If you decide to drink, choose carefully, and limit the amount you have. Current Australian guidelines for healthy adults are no more than 10 standard drinks per week, and no more than four drinks in any one day.

Best choices – dry

- dry wine – red or white – but not sweet varieties (so avoid Moscato or Riesling, fortified after-dinner whites or Botrytis)
- whiskey and brandy, and clear spirits like vodka, gin, rum and tequila – have them straight, or with ice, water or plain soda.

What to avoid – sweet

- 'alcopops' and any premixed, ready-to-drink alcoholic drinks. Although they often have relatively low alcohol content, they're very high in sugar
- sweet wine (especially many white and rosé varieties)
- most sparkling wines
- spirits when served with soft drink mixers
- beer, unless it's 'light' beer, with lower alcohol and fewer carbs
- cider
- most liquors and cocktails, including ones made with fruit juice.

---

[40] Of the five original Blue Zone groups, only the Loma Linda in California did not drink alcohol.

Fake it (at least sometimes)

It's increasingly easy to go alcohol-free. Not only is there a growing movement of non-drinkers, or people who regularly do 'Dry July' or other fundraisers, there's also an increasing range of interesting non-alcoholic drinks. You don't have to front a social event armed with no more than soda and a twist of lime. Just watch out for added sugar. Check the label and if you're mixing, use water, soda or ice.

HABIT HELPERS – REDUCE ALCOHOL

Re-think the drink. Substitute water! Plain or sparkling, with a squeeze of lime or lemon to liven it up if you like. Put it in a pretty glass, or drink it with a straw.

Adopt an AFD. Commit to having at least two alcohol-free days (AFDs) per week. If this seems too much of a stretch, start with one. Make it a regular day, and stick to it.

Treasure your body. Not drinking alcohol, or limiting yourself to just one drink, will support your beautiful, strong body.

Say it. '*I'm not drinking tonight.*' '*I don't drink during the week.*' '*I've had enough, thanks.*'

REFLECTIONS

- How much alcohol do you have per week? Per day? What strategies will you use to reduce the amount of alcohol you have overall?

- What sort do you normally have, and what do you know about its sugar content?

- If you have beer or sweetened drinks, could you change to lower-carb choices? How will you reduce or remove sweetened mixers?

Recap – What to drink

What's the problem? Most of us don't drink enough water.

Keep it close. Fill up two large bottles of water and keep them close to you during the day. Make sure they're empty by mid-afternoon.

Keep it clear. Aim for urine that's a pale straw colour.

Don't count the bonuses. Have a couple of glasses of water when you're having coffee or a meal out. Don't count it towards your target, but treat it as a bonus.

If in doubt, drink. Drink water if you're not sure whether you're hungry.

Green is good. Drink green tea, it's amazingly good for you. Have it mostly in the morning, to avoid interfering with sleep.

See through it. Soft drinks, sports drinks, fruit juices, flavoured milk – too much sugar, disguised in 'healthy' or 'fun' packaging.

Reassess and reduce alcohol intake. Aim to go alcohol-free at least a couple of days per week.

CHAPTER SIX

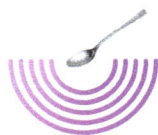

HOW TO EAT

It's common to eat without really noticing that we're eating. We often do it alone, or mindlessly, our thoughts elsewhere. And we often do it too quickly; we're in a hurry to get on to other things. We neglect to acknowledge the deep significance of what we feed our precious selves, and how we eat it. What it costs the earth to sustain us.

There are two reasons why eating the *right way* is vital for weight management. Eating without paying attention undermines our mental and physical health. It also tends to result in eating too quickly, leading to overeating and poor digestion (particularly of carbs).

In this chapter, we talk about *savouring food*:

- *Enjoy what you eat* – pay attention to food, and acknowledge its significance in your life

- *Practise mindful eating* as a technique to enjoy food more, and also to prevent overeating

- *Chew slowly and thoroughly*, and allow time for your brain to tell you when you've had enough

- *Keep a journal*, at least for a little while, to help you understand more about your own eating habits.

Savour it

Food is precious.

At its most basic level, eating is primarily a gift to our body; it's what keeps us alive and healthy. Yet it can just as easily be the opposite. Eating poorly or overeating are real threats to our health and well-being, and they're also threats to our planet.

Gratitude

Food is a gift from the beautiful, generous Earth. If we eat meat, it's also the life of another being.

Consider those who grew, harvested and transported your food. Those who prepared it for you to buy, whether from a supermarket or farmers' market. And consider those who prepared it for you to eat – maybe a cafe or fine restaurant, or someone who cares for you. Or you, for yourself.

If you have the support of others in the household, a ritual like a short prayer or acknowledgement is a beautiful way to begin meals with a sense of gratitude and mindfulness.

The first taste

Like many people, I seldom *really* thought about what I was eating. That changed a few years ago.

After becoming ill one Christmas, I ended up in a hospital high dependency unit, a mask on my face, plugged into an oxygen machine. Fever sapped protein from my muscles. The sicker I got, the less I ate.

When I returned to the general ward, peeling an orange left me too exhausted to eat it. I'd peel, then put it aside and come back later. Eat half.

When I was a bit stronger, a dear friend brought me soft-boiled eggs. When I bit in to the first egg, it was as if I tasted

---

food for the first time. The smooth, cold white; the creamy, slightly salty yolk. Remembering that moment still makes me weak with gratitude – for the egg, for Milly, and for food generally.

I try to remember to keep that feeling fresh, a reminder that food is a gift.

Overeating

It's a sensitive topic, but overweight has a lot to do with overeating – eating more than our body can use. There are numerous reasons for overeating, and none of them have much to do with moral virtue. They range from extreme genetic disorders that cause a person to be constantly ravenous, through to far more subtle emotional or habitual reasons.

One insidious reason for overeating is the sheer availability of food, coupled with the determination of food manufacturers and their advertising firms. More than 30% of all people in the world don't have secure access to food, yet at the same time we are in the midst of the opposite epidemic, with more than two thirds of all Australian adults, and a quarter of children, being overweight or obese.

Eating less doesn't achieve redistribution to those who need it, but acknowledging food inequality reminds us both to be grateful that most Australians don't suffer significant food insecurity, and to push back against forces that try to burden us with overeating.

Acknowledging food inequality also helps us think differently about food wastage. Eating more than our body needs is a waste of food, in the same way as throwing food away. Eating more than we need puts an unnecessary additional strain on ourselves, and on the Earth.

Environmental impacts of eating

Processed food 'costs' more than unprocessed food

Food production is the largest single cause of environmental degradation globally. The more people there are, the more land must be cleared and farmed to feed us.

Every item of food comes at a price to the environment – but the more food is processed, the more costly it is. 'Ultra-processed' food is the most costly and dangerous of all – yet it's cheap, cheerful, and everywhere.

How come it's so cheap? Someone is paying, of course – the Earth in general is paying, farmers of low-value crops are paying, farmers' families and local communities are paying. And in one way or another, we all are paying – with our health and our planet, if not with our wallets.

Manufacturing highly processed food uses more of just about everything: more water, energy and chemicals. Greater areas of land are now turned over to crops destined for production of highly processed food. Intensive agriculture, especially from single-variety crops, squeezes out local biodiversity. And clearing native vegetation to grow these crops drives harsh losses of habitat and wildlife. The International Union for Conservation of Nature Red List of threatened species estimates that 80% of plant and animal extinctions are driven by agriculture.

Averaged across Australia, about 40% of total calories come from ultra-processed food, and most of this is so-called 'discretionary' food – otherwise known as junk food, or in this book, *filler food* – *high-sugar and danger zone food*. It accounts for about one third of our diet-related agricultural land and water use, of our energy use, and of our CO_2 emissions.

We'd do the planet a huge favour if we drastically reduced food waste, improved food production, and ate less processed food.

According to a landmark report published by *The Lancet* in 2019 on sustainable food systems,[41] we should be eating:

- a greater variety of plant-based food, especially nuts, fruits, vegetables and pulses, and less animal-sourced foods

- more fats from vegetables, and less from animals

- only very small amounts of refined grains, highly processed foods and added sugar.

HABIT HELPERS – SAVOUR FOOD

Know where it came from, and at what cost. Be aware of the origins of what you eat. Be aware that especially for packaged food, the true costs probably aren't built into the price you pay over the counter.

Go natural. Increase unprocessed foods in your diet as much as you can, especially plant-sourced foods.

Waste not, waist not. Acknowledge overeating as a form of food wastage (and body 'waistage').

Mindful eating

We eat for all sorts of reasons that aren't necessarily associated with hunger. In earlier chapters, we looked at the importance of understanding why we eat (including our obesogenic environment), and of recognising and responding to hunger and satiety. Mindful eating takes these ideas further, and is a deliberate habit we can develop as an antidote to the eating triggers that may be sabotaging us.

---

[41] Willett (2019) Food in the Anthropocene: The EAT-Lancet Commission on healthy diets from sustainable food systems.

Eating mindfully

Mindfulness is the art of being 'present'; being fully aware of each moment. Mindfulness as a practice has its roots in Buddhism, but is now widely used in business, education, self-help and medicine as an effective method for finding calm and the many benefits associated with that: stress relief and better sleep, improved relationships, greater ability to focus, and better general health.

Mindful *eating* applies the practice of mindfulness to the specific act of eating. It means simply paying real, close attention to all of the physical, mental and emotional aspects of the act of eating, without judgement.

At a broader level, though, mindful eating also encompasses other practices that are part of the Five for Life approach. This includes being non-judgemental and loving of oneself, recognising eating triggers other than hunger and becoming aware of mind*less* eating, recognising hunger and eating only until satiated, minding portion sizes, and eating slowly and with attention. A recent study even included practices such as reading nutrition labels as an aid to mindful eating.

Research into mindful eating over the last decade demonstrates that it's an effective way to change eating habits and behaviours, which we know are the essential components of safe and permanent weight reduction. A recent controlled study neatly illustrated a direct link between specific mindfulness interventions and weight reduction. The study, reported in 2018, involved 64 participants; half of the group received a 15-week course on mindfulness as it related to healthy eating and physical activity, while the other half were a control group who did nothing different. After the first group finished the course, the control group also did it. The results for both groups after completing the course were the same: a significant increase in awareness of eating, and an average weight reduction of nearly 2 kg. All without 'dieting'. [42]

---

[42] Dunn (2018) Mindfulness approaches and weight loss, weight maintenance, and weight regain.

Changing the way we think about food and eating is the only way to achieve permanent change in our eating habits, which is the essential foundation for safe, long-term weight management.

Putting it into practice

While there are different ways to apply mindfulness practices to eating, the central ideas are much the same.

Can you remember your last meal? Exactly what you had, what it looked like, tasted like and felt like? Where you were, and how you felt, while you were eating? Chances are – not really. Next time you eat, try out the following *mindful eating method*. Aim to use it at least once every day.

Be here, now

Simply take a moment. Take a deep breath, hold it for a moment, and let it gently out. And again. And once more.

Be curious

Notice why you're about to eat. Notice, but don't judge. Are you hungry? Or do you recognise another eating trigger, such as stress, anxiety or boredom? Make a conscious, kind decision about whether you will eat, and the reasons why.

Be compassionate and grateful

Eating is an act of self-care. Consider, with gratitude, that you're about to eat. Be grateful for the food itself; for the plants or animals that produced it, and the people who prepared it (including yourself).

Set your intention

Before you take the food, set your intention: to eat only until you are no longer hungry. Estimate an amount you think will meet about 80% of your appetite and put just that much on your plate.

If you're not eating for hunger, take only the amount that allows you to savour the flavour, perhaps just a couple of mouthfuls.

Pay attention

Eating mindfully means really knowing that you're eating. Paying full attention to your food – what it looks like, smells like, tastes like and feels like inside your mouth, and as you swallow.

Take it slowly, and let this food nourish you.

Eating in the right place

Eat in a place where you will enjoy and pay attention to your food. You can't eat mindfully if you're driving the car, or sitting at your desk watching the screen, reading documents or checking emails, or while you're on the phone or watching TV. You can't focus on your food while you're walking.

So. Stand, or sit, in a place where you can focus on your food. Pay attention to it as you eat.

HABIT HELPERS – EATING MINDFULLY

Kindness. It's all about taking care of your own self; being aware of what your body needs, and how it responds to food and eating.

Support. Habit helpers in previous chapters all support a mindful approach to eating: thinking about your personal eating triggers and acknowledging them with love and forgiveness. Listening to your body when you eat. Recognising the value of what you eat, and the effects of different types of food on your body. Making choices that support your beautiful, faithful body.

Once a day. Practise the *mindful eating method* for one meal every day. It will come more naturally each time.

Remember, remember. Before you eat, take a moment to specifically visualise what you have already eaten or drunk today, including milky coffee or tea.

REFLECTIONS

- What meals or snacks do you tend to eat without thinking? Without really registering that you've eaten at all? Where does this usually happen? (At your desk, in the car…?)

- Is there a place where you eat that you feel relaxed and focused on your food? Can you regularly eat more meals in that place?

- Do you have a family tradition of acknowledgement before meals? Is it something that might benefit your own household? Or something that you could do just for yourself?

Chew!

Chewing is the physical part of eating the right way. Sounds a bit strange, because of course we chew. But most of us don't even think about or notice the fact that we're chewing, and we're unaware of the *way* that chewing properly supports our ideal weight.

Slow eaters carry less excess weight

Observational studies show that slow eaters, who chew thoroughly, *tend to be leaner than fast eaters*. This doesn't mean that some fast eaters aren't also lean, or that all slow eaters are lean. But it's a fact that lean people are more likely to eat slower than heavy people. It's also a fact that slow eaters tend to eat less at each meal. Studies show that rapid eating, on the other hand, contributes to overweight and obesity, and is associated with increased risk of developing type 2 diabetes and metabolic syndrome.

Why is this? It's probably a combination of the reasons shown in the studies, namely that chewing slowly and thoroughly:

- helps digest food properly. Good digestion ensures that we get all possible nutrients out of our food, which in turn means our body will function as it is supposed to

- increases the calories we burn to digest food (diet-induced thermogenesis)

- helps prevent overeating. Eating slowly helps us feel full earlier, as our body has a chance to register that it's had enough

- helps to change our thoughts and feelings about food and eating, for the reasons we looked at in the previous section on mindful eating.

Chewing improves digestion

We don't chew just to get the food into small enough pieces to swallow, but also to begin the chemical process of digestion. Our saliva is full of enzymes, which help break down food into particles that our body can use. One of these, amylase, is essential for properly breaking down carbs.

Chewing well allows enzymes to penetrate the smaller pieces of food, starting in our mouth and continuing through our stomach and intestines.

Chewing burns calories. More chewing burns more calories.

The process of digesting food requires energy – from chewing right through to the other end. The heat generated from breaking down the macronutrients we eat is known as diet-induced thermogenesis.

Chewing is the beginning of the digestive process, and just the simple act of chewing has an identifiable effect on thermogenesis. Studies show that the more thoroughly we chew, and the slower we eat, the higher the diet-induced thermogenesis: the more energy our body uses. The increase is only small (probably around 3% more per meal), but worth it, as supported by the observation that slow eaters tend to be leaner than fast eaters.

Adopt slow eating as an every-meal, every-snack habit – it will make a real and permanent difference over time. Chapter 7 has more about thermogenesis and the role it plays in maintaining healthy body weight.

Chewing well helps prevent overeating

The more we chew, the less we consume in a meal; studies show this can be a reduction of up to 12% in a meal.[43]

Part of the reason for this is that truly savouring food – tasting it, feeling it – plays an important role in regulating how much we eat. Another reason seems to be that eating slowly suppresses the appetite-stimulating hormone ghrelin.

We can use mindfulness practice to train ourselves to eat more slowly, thereby reducing the amount we eat.

There's a trick our body tries to play, though: when we eat food we really like, we tend to eat significantly faster. If the food you've chosen is something you particularly enjoy, be aware of this and take extra care. Set your intention for that meal or snack – to truly savour every mouthful, chewing it long and slowly before it leaves your mouth.

> ## HABIT HELPERS – CHEW YOUR WAY TO HAPPY WEIGHT
>
> ***Take your time.*** Allow each meal to last at least 20 minutes. Chew thoroughly, thoughtfully, and frequently. Put cutlery down between mouthfuls as a mental reminder to really savour the food. Practise being the last, or nearly the last, to finish your meal.
>
> ***Tiny tastes.*** Take smaller bites. Using smaller cutlery will help you do this. Use chopsticks for the ultimate in slow going!

---

[43] Argyrakopoulou (2020) How important is eating rate in the physiological response to food intake, control of body weight, and glycemia?

Chew 'til smooth. Chew until there are no more lumps. This is *at least 30–40 times*. For food with a heavy texture (e.g. steak and other cooked meat, or fibrous vegetables like kale) it might be more like 50 times. Seriously.

Tasty tempters. Look out for tasty food – our natural inclination is to eat it more quickly. Be aware, and slow it right down.

REFLECTIONS

- How would you rate your own eating speed? Are you the first or last to finish a meal? Or somewhere in between?

- How many times do you chew each mouthful? Estimate, then check next time you eat!

- What methods will you try out to eat more slowly, and chew more thoroughly?

Register it

It's common to eat without noticing, and afterwards to barely remember what we've eaten, and the fact that we're no longer hungry. This is partly due to the modern pace of life (lunch *hour?* Who even still has one? And how often is it actually used to eat, rather than do other things, such as errands or chores?). But rushing meals is also largely to do with habits.

We need to find changes in our own lives to prioritise eating meals calmly and consciously. The mindful eating exercise earlier in this chapter will help form new habits to strengthen mental and physical connections with food and eating. Another way to build better awareness, strengthening mindful eating and highlighting where you might need to focus new habits, is to write about it. Yep, a food journal.

Food diary vs. journal

It's common for dietitians to suggest that clients keep a food diary, at least in the early days. You write down everything you eat, then trawl through it with the dietitian at your next appointment.

Recording *what* we eat is a useful way to identify trends that are undermining our efforts. For example – are our portions too big? Are we eating a lot of sugar or filler foods or drinks? People also sometimes find that keeping a food diary motivates them to eat healthier food, or to eat less overall.

For some of us, though, a food diary is just an unwelcome reminder of everything we feel we're doing wrong.

Keeping a food diary

If you're interested in keeping a food diary to help identify what you're eating, and whether this aligns with the 'eat the right food' advice in Chapter 4, keep one for just five days, including both work and non-workdays. Repeat it every six weeks or so, to check how you're going.

It's a surprisingly difficult task (so be gentle with yourself); partly as it's easy to forget what you've eaten unless you enter each item immediately (not always convenient!), but also because estimating portion sizes is tricky. Use comparisons which mean something to you, for example 'one cup' or 'one large handful' or 'the size of my palm/fist'. The precise amounts don't matter as long as the estimates are consistent; you're looking for change over time.

I've created a downloadable food diary template for you, available on the Five for Life website.

Keeping a journal

Food diaries cover only the 'what' part of the eating picture. There's much more to the story – the *how and why* of eating: *your eating habits*.

For this reason, I recommend using a journal. This can include a record of what you ate, but also focus on the more subtle aspects of eating. ***Why, when, where, how, and who with?*** These sorts of details will help identify why you're not shedding kilos, or why your weight might be increasing. They can help you see when and why you're likely to eat when you're not hungry, or to eat unhelpful food, or too much of it.

Give yourself just 10 minutes at the end of each day to record your eating. Record what you ate, and a guess at how much, but more importantly, make a note of all the other aspects of eating.

Write as much as you can remember – look for clues about how your eating habits might be undermining you, or how your habits are changing. All the little details count – what you had, who you were with, how you felt, why you chose what you did, whether you enjoyed it, how you felt afterwards… If you did any food shopping, make a note of whether you were triggered by things you saw, and what you did about those feelings.

The key with journaling is to do it with kindness and non-judgement. It's an extension of the practice of mindfulness, to be done with a curious and compassionate mind.

HABIT HELPERS – REGISTER IT

The written word. For five consecutive days each month, write down the why, when, what and how of your eating, to help track your use of the Five for Life habits over time.

Recap – How to eat

What's the problem? Eating without awareness is a common habit, and it undermines healthy eating.

What to do about it? Work on changing the way you think about food and eating, including with a regular mindful eating practice.

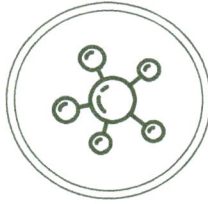

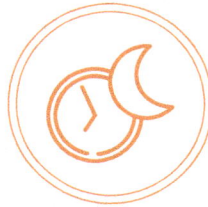

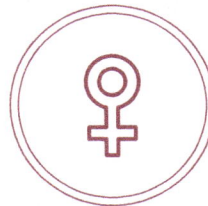

CHAPTER SEVEN

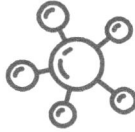

MICRONUTRIENTS, MICROBIOME AND METABOLISM

This chapter looks at the 'three M's' that influence our weight and overall health:

- *Micronutrients* – vitamins and minerals we need only in small quantities

- *Microbiome* – the tiny bugs that live in our gut and have a huge impact on our health, including our weight

- *Metabolism* – how much energy our body burns. It's key to how we regulate body weight, and there are things we can do to boost it.

Micronutrients

What are they?

Vitamins, minerals and trace elements

Vitamins, minerals and trace elements are the nutrients we need only in small amounts – this is why they're known as 'micro-nutrients'. There are about 30 different micronutrients, and our body must have them all in the correct amounts to be able to function.

Vitamins

B-group vitamins and vitamin C
These are 'water-soluble' vitamins that can't be stored in the body, so we need them from our diet every day, and throughout the day.[45] Vitamins B and C protect cells from damage and help make red blood cells; they're also needed by our body to make energy. All the B-group vitamins are essential for brain health.

Vitamins A, D, E and K
These vitamins are stored in our liver or fat cells. Among their many other functions, we need them for our immune system, including to produce antioxidants to fight inflammation.

Minerals
We need a range of minerals including calcium, magnesium, phosphorous, potassium and sodium. Their many functions include maintaining healthy bones and muscles (including our heart!).

---

[45] The one exception is vitamin B12, which we do store, mainly in our liver. Non-vegans generally have about three to five years' worth of vitamin B12 stores. If we eat no animal products, our stores become depleted, and we need to supplement.

> **Trace elements**
> We only need a very small amount of the trace elements, including zinc, selenium, iodine and copper. Trace elements act as catalysts for biochemical reactions throughout our bodies.

Polyphenols

Some compounds in food aren't technically essential for our basic function, but are still health-giving – these are plant chemicals (phytochemicals) including polyphenols, which provide antioxidant, anti-inflammatory and other benefits. Substantial evidence suggests a diet high in polyphenols protects against chronic diseases, including type 2 diabetes and heart disease, high blood pressure and high cholesterol, and potentially improves metabolism.

To increase polyphenols, simply eat more herbs and spices, tea and coffee, and vegetables and fruit, especially the colourful things.

Micronutrients in a balanced diet

It's best to get all our micronutrients from our everyday diet – a wide variety of vegetables, some whole grains, nuts, fats and a range of protein sources.

Ensuring sufficient micronutrients is another reason for never subjecting ourselves to a crash diet – any diet that cuts out food groups, or drastically reduces total energy (calorie) intake. Fasting isn't a crash diet – done properly, it can be a healthy way to reduce excess body fat. Chapter 3 has more on the difference between fasting, intermittent fasting, and potentially harmful diets.

Sometimes we need more than we get

Micronutrient 'deficiency' (not enough for your body to function safely) is rare in Australia, simply because most of us eat more than enough food overall.

Even so, many of us have what's called micronutrient insufficiency or inadequacy – we don't get enough of some of the essential vitamins, minerals and trace elements to *function at our best*.

As vegetables are our best source of many micronutrients, the main reason for insufficiency is that **most of us don't eat enough vegetables**. The Australian Institute of Health and Welfare reported in 2019 that fewer than 1 in 10 Australians eat the minimum recommended amount, which is about 400 g per day.[46]

Other reasons for micronutrient insufficiency include the following:

- Some vitamins and minerals can benefit us in doses higher than we might normally consume in our daily food. These include the **B-group** vitamins, **vitamin D**, and **iron** if you're a woman between 12 and 50 years of age.

- As we age, we need more of some vitamins and minerals. **Vitamins D** and **B**, and **iron, zinc, calcium** and **magnesium**, fall into this category.

- **Vitamins C** and the **B-group** aren't stored by our bodies, so we need adequate amounts on a daily basis.

- Some vitamins and minerals are simply more difficult to source at adequate levels in everyday food, especially processed food. It's not uncommon for intakes of **calcium, iron, magnesium, zinc** and several **B-group** vitamins to be inadequate.

- Chronic stress leads to long-term disturbances in multiple body systems, including our immune and metabolic systems. Research shows that increasing certain amino acids (which we get by eating protein), along with **vitamins B** and **C, magnesium** and **zinc**, helps to regulate the stress response.

- Some prescription medications can interfere with how we absorb or metabolise some micronutrients. For example, calcium and magnesium uptake can both be affected by proton pump inhibitors (which are used to block stomach acid) and diuretics (for treatment of high blood pressure).

---

[46] https://www.aihw.gov.au/reports/food-nutrition/poor-diet/contents/dietary-guidelines.

Vegan? Mind your iron, calcium and zinc, B12 and Omega-3 fatty acids

Vegan diets can be low in *iron, calcium and zinc,* which we need every day, so these are things to consider supplementing. Excellent sources of iron and calcium include soybeans and other pulses, broccoli, kale and nuts (particularly almonds). Pulses, nuts and seeds are also high in zinc.

Vitamin B12 isn't available from plant foods, but you can get it from nutritional yeast fortified with B12 created by bacteria. Not all nutritional yeast is fortified, so check the label.

Omega-3 fatty acids are difficult to get from plants in sufficient bioavailable forms, but there are Omega-3 supplements made from algae (kelp).

You can find a wealth of information online about healthy vegan diets. Some government websites have good introductory material, but for more detail, check out one of the many others. Sites run by dietitians with a special interest in veganism, or by individuals with a scientific and research bent, are good resources.[47]

Minerals — some of the 'big ones'

Some minerals we need in relatively large amounts each day: sodium (salt), chloride, potassium, phosphate, sulphur, calcium and magnesium. Although we generally get enough of most of them, many of us don't have sufficient calcium or magnesium.

Calcium

We need calcium for numerous processes, especially for our bones, muscles and heart. Calcium is laid down in our bones and teeth as we grow, peaking right after our teenage years. It remains at fairly stable levels until we're about 50, then begins to fall – and with it, our bone density. Low bone density (osteoporosis) is a particular risk after menopause.

---

[47]   I like https://veganhealth.org/ and https://vegfaqs.com/.

We need to top up calcium *every day*, as we lose it through urine and sweat. Good sources of calcium are milk and cheese, brassicas (e.g. cabbage and broccoli), nuts and soybeans. Many people also enjoy the subtle crunch of sardine bones, an excellent calcium source.

If you take calcium supplements, avoid having them at the same time as magnesium supplements, as these minerals block one another's absorption.

Magnesium

Magnesium is one of my personal favourites. It's essential for more than 300 different biochemical reactions, including:

- making protein for muscles and other cells

- making bone tissue and reducing the risk of osteoporosis

- maintaining a healthy heart, including by ensuring conduction of electrical signals

- maintaining normal blood pressure

- producing energy by activating adenosine triphosphate (ATP) cells (our internal 're-chargeable batteries')

- controlling blood sugar and reducing the risk of insulin resistance

- maintaining our nervous system.

Our body doesn't store magnesium, so it needs to be a part of our *daily diet*.

Up to 60% of the population in places with mostly Western-style diets, including Australia, are likely to lack sufficient magnesium. The magnesium content of processed foods is very low, so as we eat more processed food products and fewer green vegetables, our dietary intake of magnesium decreases. Diets high in caffeine, alcohol and soft drinks, and low in protein, put us at special risk of magnesium insufficiency. And simply getting older, especially post-menopause, is another risk factor.

Increase your natural intake of magnesium by eating more leafy greens such as kale and spinach, collard greens and mustard greens. Avocados, nuts and seeds (especially almonds, cashews, and pumpkin and chia seeds) and pulses are also excellent sources.

Magnesium supplementation can help to relieve anxiety and depression and modify the effects of chronic stress; it can also help relieve muscle tremors and cramps, migraines, insomnia and fatigue, and is also a great antidote to constipation. The recommended dosage is around 300–400 mg per day.

Speak to your doctor before taking magnesium supplements if you have kidney problems, and also to check for potential interactions with other medication you may be on.

FAQ — Is the nutrient content of fruit and vegetables declining over time?

There has been some debate about whether vegetables and fruit are lower in nutrients than, say, 50 to 80 years ago. The best current evidence is that *yes, there are some changes,* but these are both decreases *and increases* in various minerals and vitamins.

Copper, calcium, sodium and magnesium have generally decreased a little in vegetables, along with iodine and selenium. However, the changes are very small, and likely to be insignificant in terms of dietary intake – *provided you eat enough vegetables to begin with*!

The research theorises that changes are likely to be due to factors including differences in the type of plants studied; where and how different samples were grown; the specific cultivar or species and the time of year they were harvested, as well as other factors like the techniques for analysing nutrient values. Studies found that higher yield (usually because of changes in plant varieties, for example more tomatoes per plant) was often associated with decreased mineral content.

> Soil mineral levels don't seem to be the culprit – studies have shown no consistent evidence of depletion, with some studies indicating soil levels of nutrients have increased from historical samples.[48]

Overdoing it

If you have a chronic illness, particularly chronic kidney disease, don't take vitamin or mineral supplements, including magnesium, without first consulting your doctor.

For most vitamins and minerals, you'd need to significantly exceed the recommended dose before causing harm. (For example, vitamin B6 exceeding 1 g/1,000 mg per day for long periods can harm our nervous system.) Always check the label and take only the recommended amount.

Some vitamins and minerals we only need in tiny amounts. There's a real risk of overdoing these if we take supplements, especially if we're having multiple different supplements that might all include small amounts of these substances. Be careful with these ones in particular:

Vitamin A – too much can cause headaches, weaken your bones and damage your liver, cause nausea and even death; an excess during pregnancy can cause birth defects.

Vitamin D – exceeding the recommended dose long term can lead to heart problems. Vitamin D is currently a popular supplement, and already added to some food (e.g. margarine). A blood test can show if you're lacking vitamin D.

Vitamin E – in very large doses, vitamin E can prevent proper blood clotting and cause haemorrhaging or stroke.

Iron – too much iron can damage the liver or other organs, and cause nausea and vomiting.

---

[48] Marles (2017) Mineral nutrient composition of vegetables, fruits and grains: the context of reports of apparent historical declines.

Selenium – too much selenium can cause fatigue, brittle nails and hair loss. One or two brazil nuts per day contain an ample dose.

Drug interactions

Some vitamins or minerals can interact with prescription drugs. It's important to make sure your doctor knows what supplements you take when prescribing any new medication. And if you start taking supplements while already on prescription medication, let your doctor know.

Some important ones are:

St John's Wort interacts with many other drugs, including anti-depressants and contraceptives.

Vitamin K can reduce the effectiveness of blood-thinning medication.

Antioxidant supplements, like Vitamins C or E, can interfere with some chemotherapy medication. Vitamin C can also increase the absorption of iron, which can be dangerous for people who have the condition hemochromatosis.

Magnesium can reduce absorption of antibiotics and anti-osteoporosis medication. If you're on this medication, take your magnesium supplement at a different time of day.

Some medications can also interfere with absorption or storage of certain vitamins and minerals. One example is proton pump inhibitors (prescribed antacids), with a number of studies showing increased risk of iron and magnesium deficiency with longer-term use of PPIs.

The bottom line on micronutrients and supplementation

The subject of micronutrients is enormous, complex and still being explored.

In short, it's always best to get what we need from natural sources in our everyday diet. However, if (like many of us) you live a highly stressed lifestyle, you might benefit from extra:

- magnesium
- B-group vitamins
- iron, especially if you're a young woman
- zinc, especially if you're older
- calcium, especially if you're a woman.

As individual needs and recommended dosage vary, if you think you might be deficient in any vitamin or mineral, or could benefit from a boost, consult a dietitian or nutritionist about your specific circumstances. And importantly – talk to your doctor about the effects of your prescription medication, including whether it might interfere with uptake of nutrients.

Gut microbiome

What is it?

Our gut is full of cells that aren't strictly speaking ours – bacteria, archaea, viruses and fungi. We harbour trillions of these 'foreign' bodies – at least as many as our own human cells.[49] Together they're known as the gut microbiome – a universe of tiny things.

We each host these minute life forms (microbiota) in different numbers, varieties and proportions. What exactly is living in our own gut depends on factors including age, sex, genetics, stress, nutrition and diet. *Some of these factors we can't change, but the last three we can – and do – for better or worse.*

---

[49] For a long time, we were told that there was anything between 'twice as many' and '10 times as many' cells in the microbiome as human cells, but it turns out there are likely to be *about as many* non-human cells as human cells.

Role of the gut microbiome in our weight

What are all those microbiota doing hanging out in our gut, anyway? We aren't 100% sure what they're up to and how, and it's a rapidly developing area of research and knowledge, with thousands of studies on the gut microbiome being published in the last few years.

What we do know is that gut microbiota play important roles in fermenting and digesting food, harvesting energy and absorbing nutrients. We need them. But if they're out of balance, things can go badly for us. Biota imbalance (known as dysbiosis) is linked to a surprising range of diseases, from depression and heart disease to obesity and metabolic disorders.

We also know that healthy weight people have what is called a 'lean-type' gut microbiome, while people with overweight or obesity have an 'obese-type' microbiome. An obese-type microbiome has lower total numbers of good gut biota, and also lower overall *diversity* of microbiota. The exact mechanisms by which dysbiosis causes or contributes to obesity is the subject of ongoing research.

Creating a 'lean-type' microbiome

One thing at least is clear from the research: that to maintain a healthy weight, it's important to keep our gut microbiome happy.

It's also clear that **what we eat changes our gut microbiome, with profound effects on our health**. A high-sugar diet, in particular, reduces diversity and abundance of good biota, leading to an obese-type imbalance. Our gut microbiome can also be disturbed by medication, including antibiotics and proton pump inhibitors. Although our genes also affect our microbiome, studies show that these genetic determinants (which we can't change) are insignificant compared with the impact of diet and environmental factors – which we can change.

Simple changes in what we eat help a lot: a diet that's high in fibre and fermented foods, and low in sugar, changes the gut microbiome for the better. Studies have shown that such diets are strongly associated with reduced body fat.

The gut is quick to respond to a change in diet – starting within about 24 hours!

Improve gut health and start developing a lean-type microbiome by *eating more probiotics and prebiotics, and less sugar*. It's also worth avoiding artificial sweeteners, until we know more about them, including their impact on the gut (more about artificial sweeteners in Chapter 4).

Probiotics

Probiotics are the 'good' gut microbes themselves, but we also use probiotics to describe foods or supplements that contain those microbes. Fermented food is naturally high in probiotics. Yoghurt, sauerkraut and kimchi, tempeh and miso are excellent sources. Watch out for pickled food – it hasn't necessarily been fermented. Most shop-bought pickles aren't fermented; they just contain vinegar and generally sugar too. Check the label.

Prebiotics

Prebiotics are various dietary fibres that 'feed' the probiotics. The best sources are the types of fibre found in vegetables, fruit, oats, pulses and psyllium husk.

Sugar and other sweeteners

High-sugar diets, as well as high-sugar/high-fat diets, favour the development of an obese-type microbiome, as it turns out that lean-type microbiota don't like sugar. Artificial sweeteners as well as natural intense sweeteners (e.g. stevia) have also been shown to alter the microbiome, and not in a good way.

Probiotic supplements – friend or fad?

Probiotic supplements are concentrated preparations of live bacteria – usually in powder or capsule form. The idea is they make their way to our gut to join their friends down there. Numerous brands and preparation types are available, all containing different strains and quantities of bacteria.

Probiotic supplements have been studied for their positive effect on a wide range of serious conditions from Alzheimer's to liver diseases and even cancer. In general terms, probiotics are a 'good thing', even if we don't know exactly why, what sort, or how much, is right for different individuals.

My advice on supplements:

- Don't go self-medicating with probiotic supplements if you have a medical concern – see a professional.

- If you have had a gut-disrupting event, such as being on a course of antibiotics, there's reasonably good evidence that probiotic supplements with various *Lactobacillus* strains help restore microbiota after antibiotics.

- Other than that, stick with the natural route, improving your dietary intake of fermented foods (natural probiotics) and fibre (to feed them with). It's a much tastier and less expensive route than supplements, and has the added benefit of all the other nutrients contained in those foods.

The bottom line on gut microbiome

Disruption of our gut microbiome can make us gain body fat, and developing an 'obese-type' microbiome will mean it's difficult to shed that weight.

It's a complex area of continuing scientific work, and we're just at the tip of the iceberg. One day, no doubt, there'll be microbiome prescriptions for the precise type and number of biota for each individual, including to treat overweight and obesity. But for now, to ensure a happy gut, increase your chances of becoming and keeping a healthy weight, and avoid a host of diseases:

- eat more fibre, especially from green vegetables, pulses, oats and psyllium

- eat more fermented food, such as plain, unsweetened yoghurt, sauerkraut, kefir, kimchi, tempeh and miso

- eat more foods containing polyphenols – natural substances in plants that encourage growth of good bacteria in the gut. Good sources include tea and coffee, cocoa and berries

- eat less sugar and other sweeteners

- eat in time with your circadian rhythm. There's good evidence that eating at the 'wrong time' (night-time) also disrupts our gut biota.

Metabolism

Our metabolic rate is the amount of energy (calories) we use in daily life. This is the 'energy out' side of the 'energy in vs. energy out' equation, and it has three elements:

- Energy we use just to stay alive (e.g. to breathe, keep our blood circulating and other organs functioning) – this is our **basal metabolic rate** (or resting metabolism). It makes up around *60–80% of our energy consumption.*

- Energy we use to move – this is *physical activity thermogenesis*. It depends on the amount of physical activity we do, so the amount of energy used varies greatly. Intentional exercise accounts, on average, for *up to* 10% of energy expenditure. Non-intentional exercise (movement incidental to daily living) accounts for up to 20% of energy use.

- Energy we use to digest food – this is the **thermic effect of food** (also called diet-induced thermogenesis). It uses about 10% of our energy.

The more active our metabolism, the easier it is to reduce and maintain our weight. We don't have a great deal of control over our metabolic rate, but we have **enough that it's worth paying attention to.**

Basal metabolic rate

Our basal (resting) metabolic rate makes up the largest proportion of 'energy out', so it makes sense to focus our efforts here. We can *increase* our basal metabolic rate a little, but we can *decrease* it quite a lot – something we definitely want to avoid.

What supports basal metabolic rate?

Build muscles. Muscles use energy to work! The more muscle we have, the higher our basal metabolic rate, as we burn more energy.

- Pump iron. Push weights. Do some heavy gardening. When your children are small, carry them in a harness on your front or back rather than put them in a pusher. Carry your groceries.

- Eat protein. Without protein intake, your muscles cannot grow bigger. Another benefit of protein is that it takes more energy to digest than other macronutrients; more on this in a moment.

Drink more water*.* As mentioned in Chapter 5, drinking water seems to increase our resting metabolic rate.

Get cold*.* Our body needs to work harder, and therefore uses more energy, when our environment is very cold. Some studies have shown that regular exposure to cold may translate to increased energy expenditure. So don't be afraid of the weather! It might be helping to raise your metabolism.

What reduces metabolic rate?

Dieting. Crash dieting (severe caloric restriction) and long-term fasting both significantly reduce basal metabolic rate by as much as 30%, as our body conserves energy to maintain what it thinks is its optimum weight 'set point'. Crash dieting also significantly depletes our lean muscle mass, dropping our metabolic rate even further.

Don't do crash diets. For safe and effective fasting techniques, read Chapter 3 and follow the *Five for Life Fast*.

Getting older. Basal metabolic rate naturally slows down with age. Offset this decline by increasing muscle mass. Go harder with the weights as you get older, and increase the amount of protein in your diet.

Getting smaller (and losing muscle mass). Bigger people generally have a higher metabolism than smaller people, simply because it takes more energy to keep a large body functioning. However, this is only up to a point – studies show that the difference reduces past about 65–70 kg. On the other hand, body fat burns far less energy than muscle, so a person carrying higher amounts of fat will have a slower metabolism than someone of similar size who is carrying more muscle.

As you shed excess body weight, your basal metabolic rate may drop a little, meaning your body will need fewer calories to function. Get used to eating smaller portions of the right sort of food to support yourself through this change in metabolic rate. ***Eating more protein, and building more muscle, will help to offset this effect***.

Physical activity thermogenesis

Physical activity thermogenesis is the second element of our metabolism, and includes any form of exercise. An increase in physical activity means an increase in energy expenditure. Not just deliberate physical exercise, but also the types of activities that form part of your everyday life (walking around the office, doing laundry, working on the car – even fidgeting!). So get active.

Thermic effect of food

Our bodies burn calories to digest the food we eat. Some foods use more calories to digest than others, and some eating habits can increase dietary thermogenesis too.

Eat thermogenic foods

Eating thermogenic food has only a subtle impact on metabolism, and it certainly won't achieve a change in body fat on its own.

Nevertheless it's worth adding to your collection of healthy eating habits.

Important thermogenic foods, which all have other health benefits too, include:

- *Protein.* This is the one exception to what I've just said about the subtle effects of thermogenic food. Protein has a high thermogenic effect, and it's also essential to weight management for reasons mentioned in Chapter 4. Processed carbs and dietary fat both generate up to *10 times less* thermogenesis than protein.

- *Capsaicin*, a substance found mostly in the white pithy membranes of chillies. Capsaicin's ability to increase our resting energy expenditure has been well-studied, and widely accepted.

- Some *spices*, including turmeric, garlic, ginger, black pepper and cinnamon.

- *Caffeine*, but be aware of adverse effects on stress and sleep (more in the next chapter).

- *Green tea.*

- *Fibre*.

The effects of diet-induced thermogenesis are incremental and relatively small – apart from protein, we're probably talking about 50 calories per day. That's easily negated by habits like eating too late in the evening, or eating sugar or other refined carbs.

Adopt thermogenic eating habits

Certain eating habits increase dietary thermogenesis:

- Eating most calories earlier in the day, when the thermic effect of food is significantly higher.

- Drinking water, especially cold water.

- Chewing slowly and thoroughly.

These eating habits also have other weight-related benefits – see Chapters 3 and 8 on eating in sync with your circadian rhythm, Chapter 5 on drinking more water, and Chapter 6 on eating slowly.

Exercise helps increase dietary thermogenesis too, with studies showing that people who move more use more energy to digest their food. On top of that, of course, physical activity increases physical activity thermogenesis, while more muscles increase our basal metabolic rate.

The bottom line on increasing metabolic rate

We can increase our metabolic rate. Although the effects are small, it's a real thing, and worth doing:

- Build muscle mass.

- Add high-thermogenic *foods* (especially lean protein).

- Add thermogenic *habits* – drink more water, and chew slowly and thoroughly. Allow yourself to feel the cold.

- Add more physical activity – it doesn't need to be formal exercise. Move more, stand more, get up more.

- Avoid diets that involve energy intake of less than about 1,200 calories per day.

- Most of all – remember that ***the benefits of increasing our 'energy out' are easily outdone and undone by poor habits on the 'energy in' side of the equation***.

CHAPTER EIGHT

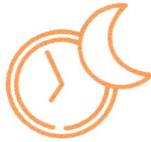

STRESS, SLEEP AND SHIFT WORK

Stress and poor sleep are potent underlying causes of excess weight. Shift work contributes to disrupted sleep patterns, and is often also combined with stress. Hence this chapter's trifecta – stress, sleep and shift working.

High levels of chronic stress and poor sleep contribute to overweight and obesity for many reasons, but they mostly come down to the function of two important hormones – *cortisol* (which goes up when we're stressed) and *melatonin* (which we need to sleep properly). Healthy levels of cortisol and melatonin are disrupted by stress, poor sleep, and lifestyles that don't align with our body clock.

In this chapter, we'll talk about the 'three S's':

- *Stress* – how cortisol affects our weight, and how to manage stress to bring cortisol levels down

- *Sleep* – why it's essential for weight management, the role of melatonin, and how to sleep better

- *Shift working* – how it wreaks havoc with metabolism, and how to use eating habits to minimise the impacts of this inherently unhealthy style of work.

Stress

Chronic stress disrupts our nervous, endocrine and metabolic systems – and these are what regulate our appetite, eating and weight. The result is that if we're under chronic stress, we're more likely to store fat, especially as visceral fat around and inside our abdomen and organs.

Stress is a normal and healthy response to danger or perceived danger and is largely controlled by the hormones adrenaline and cortisol. Adrenaline kicks in immediately our brain senses a threat. It makes our heart beat faster, pushing more blood to our muscles, ready for an immediate physical response ('fight or flight'), and it subsides quickly when the immediate threat has passed. Cortisol's role is to *keep* us in high alert, ready to maintain the fight or flight for as long as our brain thinks necessary.

How does cortisol affect our weight?

If we're in a state of constant or chronic stress, we can end up with chronically high levels of cortisol in our blood, and this has adverse effects on our immune system, digestive system and metabolism.

Long-term high cortisol levels have been shown to increase appetite for foods high in fat and sugar, such as chocolate, chips and cake. One reason for this is that such foods provide a hit of dopamine, our body's 'reward' hormone. When our cortisol is high, we seek out dopamine to help us feel better.

Research also shows that chronically high cortisol leads to redistribution of body fat to our abdominal area.

Truly a double whammy – chronic stress makes us crave the type of food guaranteed to be converted to fat, and we'll be more likely to store that fat around our middle, as dangerous visceral fat.

To help shed excess fat and keep it off, we need to drop our cortisol levels.

What causes high cortisol?

Stress – both physical and psychological – causes us to release cortisol. Chronic stress leads to chronically high levels of cortisol.

Vigorous exercise causes physical stress and does raise cortisol, but not at the exercise levels done by most people, and rarely for prolonged periods. On the other hand, moderate to low intensity exercise reduces cortisol.

So that leaves mental and emotional stress – and they're big ones. If we feel constantly under stress or threat, our bodies are likely to be maintaining chronically high cortisol levels.

Menopause is also linked to higher levels of cortisol – more about this in Chapter 9.

Manage stress

Reducing chronically high cortisol essentially means managing stress.

There's plenty of good advice around on managing stress, and certain diet and lifestyle changes can make a real difference:

- Do meditative activities every day.
- Do physical exercise that you (really, truly) enjoy.
- Spend time in nature.
- Manage caffeine and alcohol intake.
- Consider supplementing with magnesium and taurine.

It's important to talk to your doctor or other health professional if you feel stress levels are hurting your quality of life and you need help managing them.

Go within

Take up meditation or meditative physical practices like walking, yoga, tai chi or gardening.

Every couple of hours during the day, take a few minutes to just reconnect with your breath. Deep breath in, hold for a moment, and slowly, quietly release. And again. And once more.

Go fast

Getting your heart rate up with exercise that you enjoy (*while* you're doing it, not just for the after-exercise satisfaction!) improves mental health, and reduces stress.

Go outside

You might have heard of 'forest bathing' or forest or nature therapy – spending time in nature, in a green environment. Research into forest therapy began in Japan (where it's known as *Shinrin-yoku*) in the early 1980s as treatment for lowering blood pressure and cortisol levels, and improving concentration and memory. It's now part of formal Japanese Government health recommendations, and has been the subject of research in many other countries.

Not surprisingly, the research has confirmed that spending time in nature is really good for us (who would have guessed!?). Studies have linked forest bathing to decreased depression, lowered blood glucose in people with type 2 diabetes, improved sleep, reduced hypertension, lower blood pressure, lower heart rate and variability in heart rate, reduced inflammatory markers, decreased neck pain, and improved sense of general well-being and calmness. *Importantly for weight control, it also reduces cortisol levels.*

Go low

Caffeine stimulates the production of cortisol, especially in people who are also feeling stressed. Aim to keep caffeine intake below three cups per day.

Alcohol also increases cortisol release, even at low levels (blood alcohol less than 0.07%). Cortisol responses to alcohol vary a lot, increasing with factors such as higher stress levels and family or personal history of alcoholism. Dial down drinking to help reduce stress.

Consider supplements

Studies show that people suffering from high and chronic stress commonly have lower levels of magnesium and taurine. Vitamin C and B-group vitamins, as well as zinc, are also in high demand when we're stressed. While normally a good balanced diet is sufficient, when we're under chronic stress, we need greater quantities of all of these nutrients.

Magnesium is essential to our ability to deal with stress, but around one in three Australians don't get enough. Chapter 7 has more about supplementing this important mineral.

Taurine isn't commonly included in supplement blends, but we require this amino acid for a range of functions. Studies in animals, as well as recent human studies, show that it has anti-anxiety effects, including by lowering cortisol levels. Our body can make its own taurine, but only in small amounts. We can increase taurine by eating more animal protein, especially shellfish and dark poultry meat. Non-animal derived taurine supplements are available.

B-group vitamins, vitamin C and zinc are also essential for managing stress and cortisol levels. Eat more good-quality, unprocessed protein, especially salmon, beef, offal, oysters, pulses such as lentils, raw nuts and seeds, eggs and dairy for extra zinc and B-group vitamins.

Leafy green vegetables are high in vitamins B and C, while broccoli and many different types of fruit, including citrus, are high in vitamin C.

Curb cortisol cravings

It's a fact – chronically high cortisol increases our appetite for danger zone food: refined carbs prepared with fat and flavouring. Danger zone food is addictive, sparking cravings for more of it, and this is one of the key reasons why stress undermines healthy weight.

Understanding the reason for a craving can help us resist it, so if you recognise you're under chronic stress, acknowledge this might be driving a strong desire for danger zone food. Recognise it for what it is – not really a desire for these foods at all, and definitely not hunger – but a cry for a calmer life.

Take action to reduce stress, not feed it.

The bottom line on stress

Stress makes us fat. If we're chronically stressed, we're likely to have chronically high levels of cortisol. This makes us susceptible to eating sugary, refined carbs, and to storing excess fat around our middle.

Reduce cortisol levels by managing stress. Reduce sugar, caffeine and alcohol, and slow down mentally.

Build your defences. Consider supplementation, especially of magnesium and taurine.

Forewarned is forearmed. If you have a highly stressed lifestyle, recognise that this might be what's driving a desire for danger zone food.

Sleep

Sleep… one of the most precious uses of our time!

And yet, we pay too little attention to it. According to data collected by the Australian Sleep Health Foundation,[50] nearly half of all Australian adults aren't getting enough sleep, and I'm certainly one of them.

Lack of sleep contributes to weight gain and interferes with healthy weight maintenance. Our sleep cycle and circadian rhythm (internal body clock) play an essential role in regulating hormones that affect our metabolism, particularly melatonin and cortisol, but also the appetite-regulating hormones leptin and ghrelin. Melatonin works both ways, as it's also the key hormone that keeps our circadian clock running 'on time'.

---

[50] Adams (2017) Sleep health of Australian adults in 2016: results of the 2016 Sleep Health Foundation national survey.

Effects of sleep on weight

Sleep is essential for our nervous system and the way it relates to our hormonal system, including our metabolism.

Poor sleep disrupts our hormones and circadian alignment; studies show that this disruption is linked to an increase in body fat, and risk of obesity and other metabolic disorders. Inadequate sleep also increases cortisol levels, leading to increased storage of fat, especially visceral fat.

We also know from research that poor sleep causes cravings for sugary, danger zone food – such as sweets and soft drinks and refined carbs like bread, cereal and pizza. We're also much more likely to eat more overall – about 20% over our daily needs. Ongoing, chronic sleep debt also appears to harm our ability to metabolise carbs properly, raising blood sugar, increasing our risk of type 2 diabetes, and making us more likely to store excess energy from carbs as fat.

In short – improving sleep improves our metabolic health, and along with it, our ability to reach and keep a happy weight.

Improving sleep

We need around seven to eight hours' sleep every day, although that varies a little between individuals. It's natural to wake a couple of times during the night, even for just a few minutes, but we should be able to get back to sleep quickly.

Easier said than done, I know. Many people experience periods of poor sleep during their life, for reasons including poor health, anxiety or lifestyle. Difficulty sleeping is an especially common symptom during menopause (which can feel as if it goes on for decades). Part of the reason for this is that we produce less melatonin as we progress through menopause (Chapter 9 has more about menopause).

Put simply, all good suggestions for improving sleep focus on one or both of two goals:

- *Getting our hormones in the right place* – encouraging our bodies to produce more melatonin (or supplementing melatonin if necessary).

- *Getting our head in the right space* – allowing ourselves to be mentally and physically ready for sleep: relaxed, de-stressed, unstimulated, and not in the middle of digesting a large meal.

Some well-researched, practical approaches for improving sleep include:

Circadian rhythm. It's incredibly important, for weight management, sleep and general good health, that we get our body clock working as it should be. Get outside every day, during daylight hours. Try to get at least half an hour's bright daylight in the morning. Avoid light at night. Eat in a way that supports good circadian rhythm – *eat early*. Chapter 3 has more on this.

Exercise. Daily exercise, especially if it's done earlier in the day, helps the body release melatonin earlier in the evening. And, of course, exercise is a great way to release stress.

Meditation. Meditation is one of my most reliable bets for a good night's sleep. Meditating regularly brings enormous benefits to all areas of life, including better sleep. There are many apps with guided meditations specifically for sleep (I use *Insight Timer*). Great for getting off to sleep, or if you wake during the night.

Light at night. Being exposed to light before bedtime disturbs our production of melatonin. Melatonin production is triggered by darkness, and blocked by daylight and artificial light. To help melatonin do its job, avoid bright light in the hour before you go to bed. The usual suspects are implicated, of course – phones, laptops, TV, gaming. If you read at bedtime on a hand-held device, adjust the screen-settings to a dim, night-time setting. If you can, install black-out curtains or blinds in the room you sleep in, particularly if you work shifts and need to sleep during the day.

Temperature. Reduced body temperature at night helps to release melatonin, so keep the room you sleep in cool – about 18 degrees or less, a little warmer in summer months. Open the window to allow fresh air flow (but not if you'll be disturbed by outside noises).

Caffeine. Caffeine is a stimulant, so it can be hard to switch off when we still have caffeine circulating in our bloodstream. But there's another reason some people's sleep is especially sensitive to caffeine – it reduces our ability to make melatonin. So if we're already not making quite enough (e.g. because we're in menopause, or our sleep cycle is disrupted through shift work), caffeine just makes this worse. Aim to reduce daily caffeine, and cut it out after lunchtime.

Alcohol. It's fairly common to drink alcohol in the evenings, and in small amounts, it can help with sleep. But regular and frequent drinking in the evening disturbs sleep – and the more we have, the worse it is. You might well fall asleep quickly, but chances are you'll be wakeful during the night. Studies show that shortly after blood alcohol returns to zero, we're likely to wake, or have unsettled sleep: the 'rebound'. It's one reason why if you go to bed at 10 pm having had three or four drinks during the evening, you're likely to wake around 2 am.

Consider magnesium supplementation. Studies show that chronically sleep-deprived people have low levels of magnesium. Magnesium supplementation is commonly recommended for sleep, including because it can support melatonin production, and decrease cortisol levels. Check with your doctor before supplementing (Chapter 7 has more on magnesium).

Yoga. A short session of gentle yoga before bed is a wonderful way to bring mind and body back into quiet harmony, preparing us for deep sleep. It need only be 15 minutes – not a huge chunk out of your evening routine.

Melatonin supplements. For the over-55s in Australia, melatonin can now be purchased over the counter, but have a chat to your doctor about whether it's right for you. I've been using melatonin for a while, and it's had a subtle but noticeable effect.

Investigate possible underlying medical conditions

If it's just too difficult to get to sleep or stay asleep, or return to sleep once woken, talk to your doctor about possible underlying causes. These might include sleep apnoea or mental health problems. As with all health concerns, don't let it slip. Looking after yourself means acknowledging when you can't do it all alone.

The bottom line on sleep

Sleep matters. Lack of sleep disrupts our circadian rhythm and is associated with risks of serious physical and mental diseases, and an increase in body fat, especially around the abdomen.

Self-protective, not selfish. Prioritising sleep is not an indulgence, and not something that you can safely put off in the long-term. Yes, *some* people manage on very small amounts of sleep, but if your weight is suffering and you regularly feel tired or unwell, you're not one of them.

Ages and stages. Accept that what worked when you were younger might not be working any more. As we age and go through different life stages, our body's circadian rhythm changes, which means we'll respond differently to circadian disruption. This is particularly true during and after menopause.

Keep it clean. Practise good sleep hygiene; try out the tips in this section or go online for other ideas.

Shift work

Shift working isn't healthy

Shift working is associated with higher risk of disease, including cardiovascular disease, gastrointestinal disorders, breast cancer and disorders such as chronic fatigue and stress. It's also strongly linked to metabolic syndrome – a disorder characterised by a group of symptoms including high blood pressure, high LDL cholesterol, high blood sugar and abdominal obesity.

About one in six Australian employees work shifts.

How do shifts cause weight gain?

It's almost inevitable that people who do a lot of shift work will struggle with their weight. The main reason is that shift working, when it involves working at night and sleeping during the day, disrupts our normal circadian rhythm. As our body clock is responsible for regulating a host of bodily systems, it's not surprising that unsettling this internal regulation is bad for us. The more we do it, the worse it is.

Some reasons are related to the change in circadian rhythm, others not. A recent review of more than 100 scientific articles published over the last 20 years gathered a depressing list of the reasons why shift work is making us fatter:[51]

- Shift working changes our eating behaviour so that we eat meals at strange or irregular times, have only short meal breaks and are more likely to snack frequently. As we saw in Chapter 3, studies show that people with more erratic meal routines have higher risk of developing metabolic syndrome and obesity.

- It's generally difficult to get quality food during shift work, so we eat what's available – generally ending up with higher amounts of sugary carbs and fewer vegetables. We're also more likely to be influenced by what our colleagues are eating, which can be a significant factor in how and what we eat on shift.

- Eating at night-time changes our metabolism, resulting in greater fat storage (Chapter 3 has more on the circadian rhythm).

- Not having enough sleep, or poor or irregular sleep, leads to storage of abdominal fat, as we saw in the previous section. Less or poorer sleep has also been shown to cause cravings for sugar,

---

[51] Mohd Azmi (2020) Consequences of circadian disruption in shift workers on chrononutrition and their psychosocial well-being.

soft drinks and refined carbs like bread, cereal and pizza – the foods that make us fatter.

- Shift working means a longer 'eating window', as we're spending less time asleep. For example, if a shift finishes at 7 am, you might get to sleep by 9 am, and up again by 3 pm. Your eating window is the next 18 hours – at least four hours longer than it should be.

- Shift workers often report high levels of stress, which is due both to the nature of many night-roles (for example, nursing), as well as the physical stress that comes from the disruptive nature of shift work. Studies show that stressed workers have higher levels of disordered eating, overweight and obesity.

Managing weight during shift work

If you frequently work late or night shifts, or for any other reason you're up when your body would prefer you to be asleep, how can you reach and maintain a healthy weight?

First, acknowledge that it will be difficult, but it's doable. The most important thing is to plan more carefully than people who sleep during the night. Try these suggestions:

Stay regular. Set a regular meal routine and commit to it. Aim to keep the eating window short (10 hours or less).

BYO. Take your own food with you. While there might be some good workplaces out there, it's far more likely that it will be difficult to get high-quality food during your shift.

Limit what and how much. Eat only *high-protein, low-carb food after 6 pm*. Have just one small meal, or up to two small snacks, for a total of around 200 calories only. Appendix A has ideas for high-protein, low-carb snacks that are rich in micronutrients.

Drink more. Drink plenty of water during your shift. It can be difficult to drink at work if toilet breaks aren't readily available, but it needs to be a priority; plan for this as best you can.

But not caffeine... Using caffeine to stay alert during the night is likely to reduce sleep quality the next day – and poor sleep contributes to excess fat. Depending how sensitive you are to caffeine, avoid having any within eight hours of bedtime.

Watch the clock. Research into the best time to eat during shifts is ongoing, and is likely to differ depending whether you're on long-term nights or evenings, or in a frequently rotating shift. It's likely that the best advice is to time most of your energy intake for the first four hours after you wake from your main sleep, and *during daylight hours as much as possible.*

Don't cave to cravings. Look out for sugar cravings, or cravings for danger zone foods. Recognise that they're caused by the very essence of shift work – poor sleep and circadian disruption. And remember that even in your sleep-deprived, stressed or metabolically disturbed state, you still choose what you put in your mouth, and when. Chapter 10 has more on managing cravings.

The bottom line on shift working

Shift workers are far more likely to suffer metabolic syndrome, heart disease, stroke and type 2 diabetes than others. But there are things you can do to escape these risks. To successfully manage weight while working shifts, consider the points below.

Be aware of the serious health risks that come with shift working. Be aware of the likelihood of *abdominal weight gain* unless you take careful and deliberate measures, and keep them up, even when it feels as if the world is conspiring against you.

Plan ahead. It's usually not easy to find good food when you're working nights, and you don't want to leave it to chance.

Manage up. Consider talking to your work mates and leaders in your workplace about improving shift times, as well as the length and regularity of breaks.

Mind sleep and stress. Check out the tips from earlier sections in this chapter.

CHAPTER NINE

☿

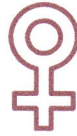

THE FEMALE FORM

It's no secret that due to hormonal and other changes, some stages of our lives are accompanied by special challenges for weight management.

Pregnancy and menopause are the most potent of these, and they predispose us to gaining fat tissue. But being *predisposed* doesn't mean that we *necessarily will* gain excess weight.

This chapter includes some tips and tricks to arm you with knowledge and the right habits to help protect healthy body composition:

- *Pregnancy* – eating best for your body and baby
- *Parenting young children* – breastfeeding, and the early years
- *Menopause* – what's going on, and what you can do about it.

Pregnancy

One of the most incredible feats achieved by the human body – to grow another human being inside it!

It's not an easy job, either, as pregnancy puts us under significant physical strain. The spaces that used to hold our own intestines, stomach, liver, kidneys, lungs and heart have to make room for a package of baby, placenta and amniotic fluid, together weighing around 5 kg by the time baby is born. Add an extra 5–6 kg of our own extra muscle mass and body fat, and it's no wonder we get so tired towards the end of pregnancy. Our heart is working overtime too, pumping up to an extra 1.5 litres of blood through our own body, and through the placenta for the baby.

Carrying all this extra weight and bulk is hard work for our lungs, heart, muscles and joints. Carrying *more than we need to* makes our body work even harder, sapping energy and reducing our physical activity. Carrying a significant amount more weight during pregnancy also raises the risk of serious health complications: gestational diabetes, type 2 diabetes, fluid retention, cardiac disease, hypertension and preeclampsia, as well as a difficult labour and greater likelihood of emergency caesarean section. It also increases our risk of remaining overweight after the baby is born, as our body will have raised its weight 'set point' (innate sense of the right weight for us) and be reluctant to bring it back down.

And it's not just about us… studies show that carrying excess weight before pregnancy, and gaining too much during pregnancy, increases the chance of passing on a risk of future overweight or obesity to our baby.

Beware the pile-on

Gaining too much weight is a common side effect of pregnancy, but *it doesn't have to be that way*. Protect yourself and your baby by using healthy eating habits to gain only the amount you need.

Gaining the right amount of weight makes it much easier to handle pregnancy, as well as the demanding days, months and years that come after the baby is born.

How much?

Your doctor, health adviser or midwife will talk about healthy weight management during pregnancy. Here are the Australian government health guidelines (single baby):[52]

- If your pre-pregnancy weight is within the low-risk BMI range, look to gain about 11–16 kg. That's about 1.5 kg by the time you're 12 weeks' pregnant, then about 1.5–2 kg per month after that (just under half a kilo per week, on average).

- If you start out in the overweight BMI range, aim to gain less – just 7–11.5 kg in total. If your BMI is over 30, look to put on only a small amount: 5–9 kg.

The Victorian Royal Women's Hospital has downloadable PDF worksheets to help track healthy weight gain during pregnancy, based on your pre-pregnancy BMI.[53]

Eat best for your body and baby

If ever there was a time to eat in a way that respects, protects and nourishes your amazing body, pregnancy is it.

We don't need many additional calories during pregnancy – we aren't 'eating for two' in the sense of greatly increasing the *volume* we have. What we do need is nutrient-rich food, high in everything that's most valuable: protein, fibre, good fats and micronutrients. We don't need filling up with empty food like white rice, bread or pasta.

Everything you put into your mouth eventually enters your bloodstream, where it's transferred to your baby through the placenta, nourishing you both. Make it count!

---

[52] See https://www.health.gov.au/resources/pregnancy-care-guidelines/part-d-clinical-assessments/weight-and-body-mass-index.

[53] https://www.thewomens.org.au/health-information/pregnancy-and-birth/a-healthy-pregnancy/weight-pregnancy#a_downloads.

What to eat

What's good for you is, mostly, good for the baby too. Focus on:

- getting **good-quality protein**
- limiting or completely cutting out food with no nutritional benefit – **danger zone food and filler food**
- drinking **plenty of water** (drinking enough can also help prevent constipation, a common side effect of pregnancy).

Additional things pregnant bodies need include:

- foods high in **iron**, such as red meat, shellfish and dark leafy greens
- an increase in **calcium** – e.g. milk, hard cheese and yoghurt. Consider skim milk to avoid excess saturated fat
- more **magnesium** – it's essential to both you and the baby, and the placenta will take what it needs for the baby from your own supplies, meaning that your magnesium requirements increase during pregnancy. Good sources are dark leafy greens, avocados, raw nuts and bananas
- more **zinc** too – seafood, pulses, milk, eggs, nuts and seeds are all high in zinc
- **DHA Omega-3** oils. We commonly don't get enough of this particular type of fatty acid in our diets anyway. Increase your intake of mackerel, salmon, flax seeds, chia seeds and walnuts, but also consider supplementing (more about Omega-3 in the box below)
- more **folate**, especially during the first trimester. The safest way to be sure you have enough is to take supplements *during the time you're trying for a baby*, and for the whole of the first trimester at least.

While it's always best to get micronutrients from a good diet, talk to your doctor about using vitamin and mineral supplements. Folate is always recommended as a supplement because of the role it plays in reducing the risk of neural tube defects.

Omega-3 fatty acids

You've probably heard that eating fish oil will make your baby smarter and healthier.

We do know that DHA, a form of Omega-3, is essential for proper brain and eye development during pregnancy and in early childhood. Some research shows that supplementing with DHA during pregnancy and breastfeeding leads to better brain development in infants and very young children, but the study outcomes are varied. Overall reviews of studies don't support a link between DHA supplementation and superior intellectual development.

So maybe not necessarily smarter – but what about healthier? There's good evidence that increasing DHA during pregnancy is likely to lead to stronger babies, with more lean muscle and stronger bones, and a lower risk of the baby being born pre-term.

The bottom line on Omega-3 supplementation

- Most of us don't get enough Omega-3 oils, especially DHA, in our diets anyway, so supplementing is helpful all round. It's estimated that only 10% of Australian women of childbearing age have enough DHA in their diet.

- During pregnancy, our own stores of DHA tend to decline as our body prioritises this important nutrient for the baby's development. (In other words – our body raids its own supplies to provide for the baby.)

- The peak body for family doctors, the Royal Australian College of General Practitioners, advises that mothers should supplement with 500–1000 mg of DHA daily during pregnancy, to reduce the risk of pre-term birth.[54] Check use-by dates, and store in a cool, dark place.

- Vegetarians can supplement with DHA from algae or kelp.

- Ask your doctor for more information.

---

[54] https://www.racgp.org.au/clinical-resources/clinical-guidelines/handi/handi-interventions/nutrition/omega-3-fatty-acid-addition-in-pregnancy-to-reduce.

What not to eat during pregnancy

- *Alcohol* – there is no safe alcohol intake during pregnancy.

- *Raw eggs* – they might contain *Salmonella* bacteria.

- *Larger fish*. Big fish such as shark (flake) and swordfish contain significant levels of mercury. Go for smaller fish like sardines and whiting. Salmon, although a large fish, doesn't have as much mercury as other large fish.

- *Food that might contain the Listeria bacteria*. Listeria infection is bad enough at any time, but can cause serious problems in pregnancy, including miscarriage. Food to avoid includes soft cheese (e.g. brie, camembert, ricotta, feta, blue cheese), sliced sandwich meats (e.g. ham, turkey slices, salami), bean sprouts, pre-prepared salad, and rice that's more than a day old (so watch out for sushi!).

Other things to avoid

Almost everything that passes into our bloodstream – including through our skin – will also pass through the placenta and into the baby, into our breast tissue and into our breast milk. So take real care with exposure to perfumes, paints and other chemicals. Avoid alcohol, drugs and all medications unless prescribed by a doctor who knows you're pregnant.

Avoid supplements containing vitamin A, as an excess raises the risk of birth defects. In Australia, most of us easily get enough vitamin A from our everyday diet.

Be supported

The advice in this section is general only, and it's important to do what's best for your own body and circumstances.

If you're pregnant or planning to be, find a healthcare professional with a special interest in prenatal nutrition, and see that person regularly.

Beware of well-meaning folk who undermine your resolve to gain the right amount of weight. You know what I mean – '*I put on 25 kg with both my children and I was fine*'; '*What are you worried about, you can eat whatever you like when you're pregnant*'; '*Come on love, you're eating for two, you know*'. Keep your eye on the aftermath. You're aiming to be strong and healthy both during pregnancy and afterwards, not carting around too much excess.

Early days, months and years

Breastfeeding

Breastfeeding is not only perfect for babies, it's also the most efficient and effective natural opportunity to shed excess fat.

Babies grow incredibly quickly, and while we exclusively breastfeed, 100% of the energy they need is coming from our own energy stores. We need on average about 675 calories per day to produce enough milk for a baby under six months of age. If we aren't eating those additional calories, then our body dips into our fat reserves for the rest, exactly as nature intended.

It's natural but... getting started

For plenty of us (including me), breastfeeding doesn't just 'come naturally'.

My advice is to set your resolve to breastfeed, and start gathering the support you need during the pregnancy. Without a solid commitment from yourself and those closest to you, it's tempting to give up when the going gets tough (and it can get really tough). Talk to your partner about it, enlist their support and line up your close friends or family too.

Contact the Australian Breastfeeding Association (ABA). They'll put you in touch with a group in your local area, where you can meet other breastfeeding mums, including plenty who've done it at least once before. They'll comfort and encourage you in a friendly, supportive environment. The ABA website has some good resources too.[55] Make the most of midwives or find a lactation consultant who can come out to your home.

Each helper will have their own advice, and their own way of explaining or showing. Sometimes that's frustrating as it can feel like everyone's telling you something different. But be confident that although there's lots of trial and error in the early days, you'll find a way that's just right *for you*.

If you can't breastfeed?

Sometimes breastfeeding just isn't possible, for all sorts of reasons.

If that happens to you – acknowledge your feelings, then let them go and move forward. There's such a smorgasbord of things to catch 'mother guilt' from, try not to make breastfeeding one of them! Infant formulas are entirely safe to use – well-researched and quality controlled. Your baby will thrive.

What to eat while breastfeeding

Our body will prioritise the baby's needs, not just for total calories, but for all nutrients. Our milk will naturally contain all the right amounts of protein, fat, vitamins and minerals, including calcium. This means we need to take special care of ourselves by ensuring we're eating enough of these nutrients.

- *Water.* Breast milk is nearly 90% water. Help maintain your supply by drinking more.

- *Protein.* Focus on keeping up your protein intake, so your body doesn't take what it needs from your own muscle mass.

- *Calcium.* If you aren't getting enough calcium, your body will rob your teeth and bones to give it to the baby. Increase your leafy greens, milk and cheese to get more calcium, and consider a supplement.

- *High-quality carbs.* Keep up your energy with some high-quality carbs – especially from those higher in protein, like pulses and quinoa, wild rice and rolled oats.

---

[55] https://www.breastfeeding.asn.au/.

Check your dietary intake of magnesium, zinc, vitamin C, D and folate, and Omega-3. Our body's demand for these micronutrients remains high during breastfeeding.

What not to eat while breastfeeding

While breastfeeding, remember that the good, the bad and the ugly all pass into our bloodstream and from there to our milk supply. Everything we put in our mouth counts. So most of all, steer clear of the danger zone foods. They offer nothing to you or your baby.

The early months and years

The pre-school years do seem to last forever, then suddenly they're gone.

Carry your babies and small children whenever you can. They're generally safer strapped to your front or back than they are in a pram or pusher. Carrying them is great for your bone strength, and for building muscle, burning up fat and increasing your metabolism. (It's also much easier to shop and get around with your hands free.) As you become stronger, they become heavier, which makes you stronger... your own tailored resistance program.

Looking after young children can be both draining and tedious. But it's still full of precious moments, even if these sometimes feel fleeting and few and far between! It helps to see the tedious, difficult bits as opportunities to do something for our own body at the same time – a chance to be more physically active. And those excruciatingly long, cold afternoons... they're a time to build our inner strength and resilience, a challenge to change our mindset by accepting the moment as it is.

Your health is never more important to you than right now. Make it an *unashamed priority* to care for yourself with eating habits that are loving and respectful of the incredible demands placed on you as a mother, both mentally and physically.

Menopause

Menopause is a topic close to my heart... and other parts of me! I'm in the midst of it while writing this book, and it's dawned on me why menopause used to be referred to as *'The Change of Life'* before people realised it's fine to give it a proper name. So much starts changing: strange aches and pains, hair loss, mood swings, thermostat malfunction – oh, and the sleep!

Certainly not everyone has a rough time of it, but it seems that plenty of us do. It can feel like it's going on forever, as changes begin in the pre-menopause stage, then progress through perimenopause, menopause and eventually post-menopause.

One of the things we may notice is how easy it suddenly seems to put on weight, especially around our middle. And how hard it can be to shift it.

But weight gain during middle age and menopause isn't inevitable, and there's plenty we can do to limit it. We can reduce the effects of hormonal changes by changing the way we respond to them. We can also be proactive about the other changes in our lives causing weight increase during this time.

What's going on?

During menopause, our body's hormone production changes. We reduce production of both oestrogen and progesterone, disturbing the delicate balance between them. We increase production of the stress hormone cortisol, and decrease the sleep hormone melatonin. There are also changes in our appetite-regulating hormones leptin and ghrelin.

Although studies so far have shown that hormonal changes may not be the direct cause of menopausal weight gain, reduction in oestrogen does change where we store the fat – typically less on our breasts and more on our bellies!

Hormonal changes also have an indirect effect on increases in weight. Lower progesterone in relation to oestrogen levels is associated with weight gain, while reduced oestrogen contributes to loss of muscle mass and muscle strength. As oestrogen helps to dampen our appetite, a drop in oestrogen can increase hunger and overeating. Increased cortisol levels, and decreased production of melatonin, are linked to increased stress and poorer quality sleep, which we know also contribute to weight gain.

And to cap it off, studies suggest that carrying too much body fat may increase menopause symptoms including hot flushes and joint and muscle pain. The good news is that the reverse also seems to be true, so reducing body fat can reduce some symptoms.

On top of the hormonal influences, there are many lifestyle factors contributing to weight gain during middle age. Menopause often coincides with higher levels of stress at work and at home, less time to ourselves as those close to us need more care, and sometimes, 'self-medication' of stress and anxiety with alcohol. We often have lower levels of physical activity than when we were younger, partly due to fatigue, but also because we tend not to prioritise looking after ourselves.

Lifestyle changes can create a negative feedback loop too. If we're emotionally and physically depleted from external demands and disrupted sleep, we're less inclined to leap out of bed at 5.30 am for a pre-work run, or go for a walk after dinner. We may be less likely to have the mental energy to prepare good meals, or instead seek meals and drinks with friends for the social boost, to relieve stress and wind down. Alcohol and late meals contribute to poorer sleep and increased fat storage, and so it goes on.

Why does it matter?

Weight gain during menopause, especially an increase in belly (visceral) fat, isn't just uncomfortable and contributing to menopause symptoms, it's also a significant risk for developing metabolic syndrome and the diseases that go with that, as well as certain cancers, including breast cancer.

Importantly, don't just trust the scales on this. *Even if our weight is in the 'healthy' BMI range, carrying too much fat puts us at significant*

235

added risk of breast cancer. Recent research looked at a group of 3,460 American women who had been followed up regularly over a period of nine to 20 years.[56] During each follow-up, body fat was measured using both waist measurement and an X-ray method known as a DEXA scan.

All participants were within the recommended BMI range throughout the study (BMI under 25), but their stored body fat varied quite significantly. The differences in breast cancer risk after menopause were dramatic. *Each extra 5 kg of body fat* increased risk of oestrogen-receptor positive breast cancer by more than 50%. Risks increased significantly as fat exceeded about 34% of total weight. And this was a group whose weight was entirely within the 'healthy' BMI.

Protect yourself from serious risk of breast cancer and keep a close eye on waist measurements, no matter what your BMI. Increase muscle mass and decrease body fat.

What can we do about it?

The way we respond to menopausal changes through our lifestyle and routine – *our daily habits* – counts for a lot. There's plenty we can do to help navigate and reduce the effects of hormonal changes on our weight and body composition.

Get physical

A large part of our increase in body fat during and after menopause can be blamed on loss of muscle (sarcopenia). It 'costs' our body more energy (calories) to maintain muscle tissue, so when we lose muscle, our metabolism slows down. Slower metabolism means the fuel we eat is more likely to get stored as fat, because our body simply doesn't need it.

Although both men and women begin to lose muscle from about 30 years of age (by as much as 8% every 10 years!), women are at

---

[56] Iyengar (2019) Association of body fat and risk of breast cancer in postmenopausal women with normal body mass index: a secondary analysis of a randomized clinical trial and observational study.

higher risk of developing sarcopenia during menopause, partly at least due to the reduction in oestrogen.

Happily, we can do quite a bit to prevent or slow down sarcopenia:

- Take up regular strength-training with weights to build muscle mass.

- Increase physical activity generally, especially walking. Carry weights while walking, using a well-fitting backpack loaded with water, or a specially designed weight belt, to increase the load and further build up muscles. Heavy gardening and yoga are also good ways to use our own body weight to maintain and build muscle mass.

- Eat more good-quality protein, such as fish, eggs and poultry, to support muscle growth. It doesn't matter how much exercise we do – *if we're not eating enough protein, our body cannot build and keep muscle.*

Improve sleep quality

As we saw in Chapter 8, poor sleep contributes to weight gain and other health problems too.

Do you fall asleep at 9.30 pm utterly exhausted, only to wake at 2.30 am? Then lie there until 4 am? This is an all-too-common part of life for many of us once we enter menopause. It's definitely one of my signature pieces, and it's really wearing. A 2016 study of Australians' sleep patterns for the Australian Sleep Health Foundation found that nearly half of all women wake frequently overnight, and that increases with age.[57]

Part of the reason is that from menopause on, women produce less of the sleep hormone melatonin. Even though this is a natural process, we can offset it a little – Chapter 8 has some tips on how to encourage our bodies to produce more melatonin at the right time.

Apart from reduced melatonin, menopause brings additional reasons for poor sleep – our thermostat playing up with night-time

---

[57] Adams (2017) Sleep health of Australian adults in 2016: results of the 2016 Sleep Health Foundation national survey.

hot flushes, and the effects of stress or anxiety. For these symptoms, sleep hygiene, reducing alcohol and caffeine, meditating and other non-pharmaceutical approaches, as well as hormone supplementation, can help.

Manage stress

Levels of the stress hormone cortisol commonly rise just before, during and after menopause. Increased cortisol affects our metabolism… and not in a good way, as we saw in the previous chapter.

Stress and cortisol in menopause is an unpleasant chicken-and-egg situation: not only do we increase production of cortisol as we age (even if we aren't feeling stressed), but menopause itself can also be a cause of stress – fuzzy head, disturbed sleep, irregular periods, joint pain, irritability and mood swings aren't much fun. And then there's the timing – menopause often coincides with added stressors of mid-life: perhaps increasing responsibility at work, difficulties at home as our children traverse late adolescence into adulthood, or ageing or sick parents, partners or pets.

Chapter 8 has more about managing stress and cortisol levels. If you're thinking about hormone replacement therapy, be aware that oral oestrogen has been shown to increase total cortisol levels, whereas transdermal delivery (patches or gel) doesn't seem to. Ask your doctor more about this.

Consider supplements

Some micronutrients, especially magnesium and calcium, can help manage menopause symptoms including anxiety, poor sleep and loss of bone density.

Herbal therapies are available, but be sure to seek out reliable advice, as only some are supported by evidence. If you decide to go this route, let your doctor know, because some can interact with other medicine you may be taking. Be aware that the quality of herbal supplements is poorly regulated in Australia, so take special care about where they're coming from and how they're made.

Foods high in natural plant oestrogens (phytoestrogens) may help some people; these include red clover and pulses, fresh soybeans and soy products such as tempeh and tofu.

Progesterone production can be supported through adequate intake of vitamins C and B6, as well as magnesium and zinc. Green vegetables, nuts, chickpeas, pumpkin, salmon and eggs are all good sources of these nutrients.

While we're on the subject of supportive diet, mind your protein intake too. Apart from being essential to maintain our muscle mass, we need protein to produce and help regulate hormones, including our sex hormones and hormones that regulate metabolism and appetite.

Hormone therapy

We can make direct changes to oestrogen and progesterone levels by supplementing through menopausal hormone therapy (MHT, formerly known as HRT). MHT usually makes a significant difference to hot flushes and sleep patterns. In terms of weight management, studies also indicate that MHT reduces abdominal fat (although not total fat), as well as having other positive effects such as reducing risk of type 2 diabetes and improving insulin sensitivity, and improving the ratio of 'good vs. bad' cholesterol.

Many women find MHT also provides effective relief of other menopause symptoms, including sleep disturbance and the odd stuff like dry eyes, hair loss and brain fog. There are many different options, from tablets to intra-uterine devices, gels, patches and pessaries, which are useful for people whose gut doesn't take kindly to digesting hormones.

Talk to your doctor about MHT if it sounds like your thing; preferably, see a doctor with special interest in menopause and pick their brains.

Join the club

If you're approaching menopause or in the midst of it, it's important to keep a positive outlook. Millions of other women are experiencing it too, so we're far from alone. Help is everywhere – from medical to allied health, to naturopathy, chiropractic and others. Find out what works for you.

Most of all – don't suffer in silence, and resist blaming your body; menopause is a natural part of our lives, and not something to punish our beautiful bodies for. Resist external pressure too. I've been surprised by how many feel that seeking help on menopause is somehow 'giving in', or giving up. It's an emotive area, somewhat like 'natural' childbirth and breastfeeding. If 'natural' works well, that's wonderful, and something to feel grateful about. But if it doesn't work for you, there's no point suffering with symptoms that may be having a profoundly negative impact on your life, if there are safe and effective ways to manage them.

The bottom line on menopause

Everyone will experience menopause a bit differently, but there's much common ground. To improve your chances of sailing through it with a semblance of grace:

Muscle up. Make building and keeping muscle mass a priority:

- eat more protein every day – a minimum of 1.2 g per kilo of your body weight (see more in Chapter 4)
- lift weights (even carrying the shopping counts)
- walk a lot.

Slow down. Manage stress – reduce alcohol, practise meditation, do other meditative activities (e.g. yoga or tai chi, art or sewing) and get out into nature as often as you can.

Read up. Learn more about menopause and what your options are.

Speak out. You don't have to do menopause alone and in silence. Talk, rant, cry and laugh about it.

PART III

LIVING THE FIVE FOR LIFE

Knowing what to do is one thing – but putting new habits into everyday practice is quite another. In this part, we'll look at how to make healthy eating habits work in daily life. How can we tackle inevitable challenges, including the things we seem to have no control over, that are undermining our efforts to eat healthily?

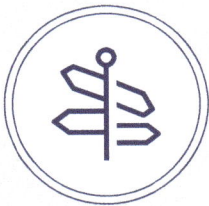

CHAPTER TEN.
NAVIGATING THE DAY

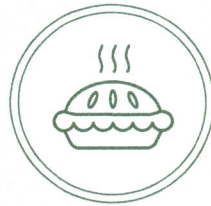

CHAPTER ELEVEN.
WHAT'S COOKING?

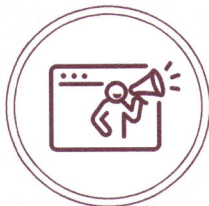

CHAPTER TWELVE.
FOOD ADVERTISING –
DON'T BUY IT

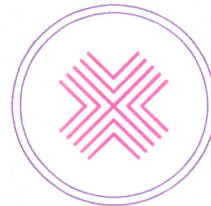

CHAPTER THIRTEEN.
THAT'S ALL FOR NOW

CHAPTER TEN

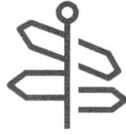

NAVIGATING THE DAY

Because eating is often a pleasure-based activity, changing the way we think and act around food can be difficult. And if our brain associates eating with a sugar hit, changing the way we eat can feel like an impossible task.

We need patience with ourselves, and with situations we find ourselves in. We also need some very practical tools.

The first step is to become aware of eating triggers that undermine our weight goals. This is where keeping a journal or notebook can be a great help. Get to know your triggers, write them down, and look out for them in everyday life. The second step is to develop strategies to swap old habits for new ones.

Earlier chapters suggested 'habit helpers' for each of the five healthy eating habits, but in this chapter we'll look at strategies to help make these new habits stick, based on three tools: *Think, say, do*. We'll also look at how to use this approach to manage some everyday challenges:

- *Workday hazards*
- *Eating out and socialising*
- *Snacking and cravings*
- *Living with younger children.*

Three tools – think, say, do

Most of the strategies in this chapter revolve around:

Things to think – change the way you think about food and eating, including by making a commitment to yourself, by planning ahead, and by anticipating and being ready.

Things to say – use your self-talk, and what you say aloud, to your advantage.

Things to do – practical responses that can become new habits, including using *substitution* to replace old habits with new ones, and *context* (time and place) to cement them.

Think

Remember habit number 1? ***Love you. Treasure your body***.

It's the fundamental element in changing how you eat. It's the reason you're doing this; the reason you'll find a way through every scenario.

Commitment

One good way to establish a new habit is to take away the element of choice. Committing to a habit by making a formal promise to yourself means it's not optional. This chapter explores a few ways to apply the idea of a promise in everyday situations.

Planning ahead

Thinking ahead about what challenges you might face in your day, and how you'll respond, is a powerful way to create your own armour; to make your own choices rather than have them made for you, or made impulsively in a way that doesn't support your weight goals.

Say

Use positive self-talk, and find ways to respond to other people if you're feeling undermined.

Sometimes it helps to remember that **we can eat whatever we like** – no one's making us do anything, and we can use self-talk to remind us. '*The only person who's in charge of what I eat is me.*'

It's not just what we say to ourselves, but also what we say to others, that helps change habits. When we make food choices that support our weight goals, it's common for others to resist or undermine that (whether intentionally or not). You know what I mean – '*Oh just one won't hurt*', or '*I'd rather enjoy my life than be worried about calories all day*'.

Answer – to yourself, or out loud if you like: '*Your choices are for you. I can eat what I like.*'

'*I enjoy my life more when I'm at a happy weight.*'

'*I don't worry about calories all day – I just choose to eat well.*'

Do

Build your own checklist of habit helpers, using ideas from previous chapters or other things you've found work for you. Each fortnight, add some new ones to the list. When you've repeated a habit helper daily for a couple of months, it's well on the way to being an everyday part of your life… that eventually you won't even need to think about.

Tactics I find useful in pretty much any situation are:

- drinking more water, or a cup of tea or coffee
- moving away from the food source – the table, the kitchen, the pantry
- doing something physical – a short walk, or five minutes of yoga or stretches, to reconnect mind and body. (Okay, so this one probably isn't going to work at a social function! But it's good for many other occasions.)

You might find it helpful and motivating to list your chosen habits as a tick-sheet and 'score' yourself at the end of each day. Keep the habits small and specific, and focus on what you *do* (not what you don't do).

For instance:

- ✓ Ate a high-protein, high-fibre breakfast
- ✓ Drank three litres of water
- ✓ Ate one meal or snack mindfully
- ✓ Met my daily protein needs
- ✓ Lifted or carried something heavy
- ✓ Ate non-starchy vegetables with at least three meals
- ✓ Finished my last meal before 6.30 pm.

Keep the habits small and easy to do, rather than going immediately for fundamental changes. If you're having trouble increasing water intake for example, first focus on that. Your list could include actions such as *'had a glass of water first thing after I got up, had peppermint tea straight after lunch, drank two glasses of water before dinner'*.

Technology can help with this – app developers have jumped on to the idea of habit-building, so there are plenty to choose from. Be aware of what the app owner can do with your data (e.g. on-sell it). If you use a habit-helping app to receive reminders and generate records of achievements, keep the number of habits small and their complexity low. Being constantly reminded of the things we haven't done can be irritating and demotivating.

Substitution

Changing habits seems daunting when we look at it only from the perspective of *'what I can't do'*. Turn this around – what *can* you do? Use **think, say, do** to substitute new routines for unhelpful ones.

Think

- Recognise the eating habit you want to change and the trigger (cue) for that behaviour. It can take a while to identify the real trigger; be prepared to do some digging.

- Choose the substitute behaviour. This can be something food-related (if the habit is about food choices), or nothing to do with food (if the habit is eating when you aren't hungry): for example, call a friend, drink tea, or do something physical.

Say

- Tell yourself about your new choice. Practise saying it in your head and out loud: '*When I'm stressed, I... have a pot of peppermint tea/take 10 deep breaths/call Annette*'. Writing it down helps too. Put it on a sticky note somewhere you'll see it.

Do

- Now practise doing it. Every time you recognise the trigger for the old behaviour, repeat the substitute strategy in your head or out loud as you do it.

My own trigger and substitute

When I'm stressed at work, I tend to hunt for a sugar hit to help me over a tricky spot. I know it.

Substitute behaviour that usually works for me is to chew on a piece of cinnamon bark or fennel seeds. They're vaguely sweet, and it involves putting something in my mouth. Consciously reminding myself that this is what I do, and keeping a small bowl of fennel beside my keyboard, helps cement my intention and takes away the 'choice' of looking for something sugary.

Context

Context – the '*when and where' of behaviour* – is a central part of all habits.

You can help a new habit stick by joining it to an existing habit that you do in the same place, or at the same time. For example, every time you get in a car, you put your seatbelt on. Use this connection to 'stack' another habit, so every time you get in a car, put on your seatbelt and... remind yourself of your compassion. That your body deserves to be treated as the magnificent miracle that it is.

Context is also part of the cement that sticks you to unhelpful habits. For example, when you shop at a particular supermarket, perhaps you always get a coffee from the place near the exit on your way out. Or you always have a biscuit with your first cup of tea at work.

Use a change in context to escape old habits. One way is to use the context as a trigger for different behaviour. For example – when I leave this supermarket I always … *focus on keeping a strong core and good posture while I carry the bags.*

Another approach is to change the context altogether. Leave the shopping centre through a different exit, change the time you shop, or shop somewhere different.

Workday challenges

Mid-morning get together or office birthday tea

Even since 2020, many of us do still work regularly in an office environment, where old habits like morning tea and birthday celebrations endure.

How to navigate Wednesday cake-day, any-occasion muffin break, or the team meeting treat?

The food on offer usually doesn't support healthy weight! It's likely to be attractive and highly sugared; it might even be a trigger food for you. Plus, there are often strong social influences – peer pressure, expectations and habits.

Do...

- Visualise the likely food, and identify whether it's highly processed danger zone material. Remind yourself *'I don't eat that any more'*, and practise supportive self-talk. *'I'd prefer not to. I take care of my body and want to be the healthiest I can'.*

- Drink a couple of glasses of water about 15 minutes beforehand.

- When you arrive, involve someone in conversation or make a cup of tea; stay back from the table.

- Acknowledge if the food is a trigger for you, and remember that this is what manufacturers want: for you to crave this, to yearn for more of it. Don't be manipulated.

- If the event coincides with your meal or snack time, eat before you turn up.

- If there are healthy choices, and you decide you want to eat, mind your portion size, as it can be easy to underestimate when taking from a platter. Put some on a napkin or plate, then move away from the table.

- Speak up about having morning teas that include cheese, nuts and vegetables.

Birthday cake tactics

There can be quite a bit of pressure to accept birthday cake. Say enthusiastically '*Looks delicious! But not for me, thanks*'. If you find yourself holding some, pass it on or put it down.

If you *choose* to have cake, have just a small piece. Pause to remind yourself why you've taken it, and to feel gratitude. Eat a mouthful, slowly and thoroughly. Taste it, feel it. Enjoy it.

There will probably be colleagues in the room who are struggling with their own weight, who might feel defensive if you turn down sugary offerings, and put pressure on you to eat with them. Be ready, as this can be really difficult. Practise saying '*no thanks*'. You don't need to justify yourself.

Lunchtime

As we saw in Chapter 3, we're more likely to reach and stay at our best weight if we have most of our food before about 3 pm. This means either making lunch our main meal, or eating two or three smaller meals during the day.

Bringing your own food to work is usually the best choice, but if you need to buy lunch out, or eat what your workplace supplies:

- as far as possible, choose an identifiable lean protein source with plenty of salad or vegetables. Beware of dressings and sauces, as they're often high in both sugar and vegetable oil. Avoid stir-fries, and pasta and rice-based salads

- the portion size is likely to be more than what you need. Be prepared to save some for later, or leave it if there's no safe storage.

Later sections in this chapter have tips for eating at restaurants and cafes, and what to do if you're caught short on choices.

Mid-afternoon low

The mid-afternoon slump is often about work burn-out, a natural 'low' in your circadian rhythm, boredom, or a combination of these. It can also be due to rebound cravings if you've had a sugar hit earlier in the day. As your habits change and you eat less sugar and refined carbs, the severity of cravings will also reduce.

This is the perfect time of day for a physical approach:

- Have a glass of water, and get up from your desk or chair.
- Then – go for a short, brisk walk.
- If you can't leave the building, do a five-minute yoga session. In just five minutes, you can reconnect your mind and body. Centre yourself. Recalibrate ready for a fresh start. You don't need to be wearing special clothes, or even leave your desk. Turn inwards, just for five minutes. Check out the internet for plenty of suggestions.
- Keep a selection of your favourite herbal teas close by. When you're back at your desk, pour yourself a cup or (better) a pot.

Stress

The first thing we tend to do when we're stressed is reach for sugar. This is absolutely me; the closer and more difficult a deadline, the more likely I am to hunt for something sweet – anything! I try not to keep sugary carbs in the house for that reason, especially if I'm going through a tough patch with work.

There may be a couple of biological reasons – first, our brains need glucose to function. When we're under acute mental stress, our brain needs 12% more glucose than in normal conditions! The quickest way to get glucose is to eat carbs; the higher the GI, the better. The highest GI foods are refined carbs including sugar and white bread.

Another reason we seek sugar is that it seems to blunt our brain's stress response – we eat sugar as a quick way to de-stress, even if it's only temporary.

What to do? Resist feeding the stress with sugar, as it makes things worse – you'll be reaching for more as soon as the effects wear off. Look for a lower GI carb, such as a piece of fruit.

Most importantly, though, learn to deal effectively with stress by using techniques such as deep breathing and mindfulness practices. Chapter 8 has more on managing stress.

Socialising

Eating is naturally a social activity, and this is something to embrace rather than shy away from. With practice, you can navigate social eating calmly and without undermining your health goals.

A couple of things will help:

- Be ready for peer pressure and expectations. Identify those who tend to undermine your determination to change your eating habits (whether they mean to or not), and the way they do it. Think of some good responses, and practise saying them aloud. Anticipating their behaviour will help it just wash over you.

- Understand your personal triggers for unhelpful food choices when you're out with friends, and work out a plan to deal with them.

Coffee morning

Morning get-togethers with friends or work colleagues, or after dropping children at school, are welcome relief from other demands on our time, and occasions we look forward to.

They don't need to include cake. Order your favourite type of tea or coffee. Be aware there's a significant amount of carbs and fat in a flat white, cappuccino or latte – around 200 ml of milk, depending on the size of the cup. If that's the way you enjoy your coffee, factor it in to your daily eating routine as the equivalent of a snack.

Get a jug of water for the table and have a couple of glasses while you wait for the coffee.

Afternoon drinks

Getting together with friends or neighbours for an easy lunch or an afternoon drink can be a lot of fun, a break from work or respite from childcare and home duties. Alcohol is often the main challenge here, along with portion creep and food quality.

Alcohol. Decide beforehand how much you'll drink, and stick to it. Drink plenty of water. Take your own sparkling water and refill your alcohol glass with it.

Portion creep. Lunches and nibbles with drinks often involve platters. It's difficult to track how much we eat when taking food from a platter. Get a small plate or napkin, and take a single serve – around one large cupped handful. Move away from the table and leave it at that.

Food quality. Typical offerings are chips, cheese or dips with biscuits, perhaps cured meats and olives. You can choose either not to eat (*are you hungry?*), or to eat. If you choose to eat, work out why you made that decision – be conscious about it, then look for the lowest sugar, highest protein food:

- Cheese. Hard cheese is best; avoid flavoured cream cheeses (e.g. the 'apricot and almond') as they're high in sugar. Have cheese by itself – leave the biscuits on the plate.

- Raw vegetables. Have plenty.

- Nuts. If they're raw and unsalted, perfect. Beware, though – nuts are often oil-roasted and salted, or presented in mixes with high-carb things like crispy rice morsels, sultanas, or chocolate- or yoghurt-coated bits. Recognise these as danger zone food and stand back.

- Dips. They're almost always high in both sugar and processed oils. Leave the dips alone unless you made them yourself and know they're low sugar with healthy fats.

Bring your own dip

A delicious and simple dip is a can of cannellini beans, a clove of garlic, lemon juice, salt and pepper, cumin and olive oil, all blended up. Serve with raw veggies or grain-free seed biscuits.

Crushed avocado with plain yoghurt, fresh herbs and lemon juice is another good one.

After the gym, yoga or bike ride

After going to the gym, or yoga session or that long bike ride, you and your mates might stick around for a while for a coffee, or lunch. When faced with the pie warmer, the cake display, chocolate bars or other triggers, it's easy to think *'I worked hard today, I deserve it/I can afford it'*.

Catch out the attitude – it's one we've been taught by sugar companies and food advertisers. Reality is…

'Deserving' it – what our body deserves is support and respect. The activity we've just done is a gift, not to be undermined. Allow the energy used during exercise to bring you a little closer to your ideal weight, not for the after-exercise snack to take you further away.

'Affording' it – what we eat is responsible for about 80–90% of our weight. It's all too easy to underestimate the amount of energy in a biscuit or a cup of milky coffee, and overestimate the amount used during exercise. For example, a small cafe latte and small muffin or cake (mostly refined carbs, sugar and processed vegetable oil), equate to at least 300 calories. You could burn that off with a 45-minute brisk walk or an hour's intense yoga lesson. But then what will burn off your breakfast, lunch, dinner, and other food and drink?

Eating out

Eating out with friends – at their house or yours, or at a pub, cafe or restaurant – is one of life's great pleasures. And of course you can keep doing that! Just plan ahead and use the other tips in this book, and you'll stay on track.

Until you reach your target weight, approach cafe and restaurant food with extreme caution. Limit how often you go, and take care with what, when and how you eat. Avoid takeaway and fast food altogether.

Plan ahead

Choose well

If you have a say in it, choose somewhere most likely to have options that will suit you. A venue that serves only pizza and pasta isn't going to help. Nor is a sushi bar, unless you only have the sashimi (raw fish, no rice).[58]

Time it right

Eat as early as you can, so you can finish at least three hours before bedtime. Go out for lunch instead, if that's an option.

---

[58] Sushi rice is prepared with a syrup of vinegar and sugar, to keep it nice and sticky, as well as flavoursome. Then there's the mayonnaise, teriyaki sauce and other treatments that pile on the sugars.

Set your intention

If you have a chance, before arriving at the venue:

- At a time when you aren't hungry (e.g. straight after lunch), go online to look at the menu.
- Read the whole menu, visualising the dishes.
- Choose from the entrée or 'small plates' list. Tell yourself aloud that's what you'll order.
- Have a couple of glasses of water before you leave to go out.

When you get there

Drinks

Drink water before you have any alcohol, and don't order soft drink. If you have alcohol, choose something with lower sugar (e.g. red wine rather than white or sparkling; light beer rather than full strength; plain spirits without a mixer, or with plain soda water).

Choose quality

Going out for a meal is usually a treat. Make it count.

Recognise 'cheap and nasty' from the menu. Avoid food that's high in starchy or poor-quality carbs (batter, dumplings, potato, rice, gnocchi, pasta and noodles), or that has been fried or deep-fried.

Look for high-quality food that your body deserves. That has been prepared with care and beautifully presented.

Quantity – one is enough

Order just one course, and if it's an evening meal, make it an entrée. If the dish you like isn't listed in entrée size, ask if it can be prepared that way.

If it looks like everyone will be having two courses and you don't want to stand out, order two entrees, or an entrée and side salad or vegetables.

Practise portion caution

If you've ordered a main course, when the meal arrives take a good look at the size of the plate and the serving, to get your bearings. Remember what an appropriate portion looks like when you serve yourself at home.

Before you start eating, divide the food, separating out a fist-sized portion. Expect it to be only around one third, or up to one half, of what was served.

Now set your resolve for this meal; an acknowledgement that the remaining portion is not necessary, and will take you further from your weight goal. Leave it on the plate, or ask for it to be packed to take away. Eventually restaurants, and other eaters, might come around to the idea that quantity does not equate to 'value', and that it is harming us.

If you have soup, ask for it to be served without bread. You don't need to add filler food to this meal.

Another way to tackle portion sizes is to share with others at the table.

Eat mostly vegetables

Order dishes that are bursting with green or brightly coloured vegetables. Avoid starchy vegetables (potato chips, corn cobs and root vegetables) and rice.

Sauces and salad dressings

Sauces and dressings in restaurants usually carry a lot of added sugar, even the savoury ones. Honey, maple syrup and similar sweeteners, even though natural, increase our blood sugar.

It wasn't until type 1 diabetes arrived in our family that we realised how much hidden sugar is in restaurant food. After years of experience, our estimates of insulin requirements for a meal are still usually too low. The safest meals have turned out to be basic pub fare – grilled meat or fish with salad and vegetables (no dressing).

Bread on the table?

Many restaurants still bring bread to the table. Leave it on the plate or in the basket. Even wholegrain, stone-ground organic sourdough is an unnecessary addition to your waistline, especially in the evening. Get all the nutrients you need from your tasty meal.

Dessert

If it looks like everyone is having dessert – be the one who doesn't.

Do the people you go out with pester you for not ordering dessert? Just like if you go cold on alcohol, cutting down sugar can make other people feel uncomfortable, as they question the way they're treating their own bodies. Remind yourself what dessert is made of, and the reasons why your brain thinks it wants some. Remember also that to make the most of your overnight fast, you need to stop eating at least three hours before bedtime.

Finishing a meal with a pot of herbal tea is a weight-friendly new habit.

Eating

Eat mindfully – take a moment before you begin. Chew slowly and thoroughly, relishing each mouthful. Flick back to Chapter 6 for more tips on mindful eating.

If your entrée serving is tinier than you expected – relax. You've just done yourself a special favour. Savour this tiny, flavoursome thing. A small meal is not something to be frightened of, or unhappy or angry about, even if you feel hungry. It's a welcome rest for your body.

If possible, move around the table to chat to people. You don't need to focus on food, or eat heavily, to get the most out of a social occasion.

Reduce the amount of alcohol you have, to support your resolve to eat in a way you'll be pleased about tomorrow.

Limit how often you do it

Eat out rarely. Until you reach your ideal weight, keep evening meals out to once a month at most. Socialise with friends in other ways – meet for breakfast or lunch, or go for a walk.

Once you've reached your target weight, you can safely increase meals out if you use the strategies in this section. The more you practise them, the more naturally they'll come to you. Keep in mind that even with healthy eating strategies, cafe and restaurant food is likely going to be higher in fat and sugar than a home-cooked meal, and will always be something to be wary of.

Between a rock and a hard place – when choices are limited

Plenty of times, I've been out on a field trip or all-day meeting, caught short on decent food options and wishing I'd thought it out better. There are two main ways to tackle this.

Fast instead

If there are no good food choices, you can choose to fast. It's an opportunity to take an unintended intermittent fast, and let our digestive system rest.

Support your choice with positive self-talk: *'If the choices aren't worthy of my body, I give my digestive system a rest. If my body needs more fuel, it will use its reserves.'*

The fasting option is fine, provided you have a plan for breaking the fast with a healthy meal. Check that your plan is feasible; it might be better to find something to eat. For example, if you won't be able to access good food before 6 pm, it's midday and you haven't had anything since breakfast, it's probably better to find something to eat.

'Better than'

If there isn't likely to be a good meal available inside a reasonable hunger horizon, I use a 'better than' approach to work out the best of the worst.

Prioritise protein and vegetables, and have just enough to keep hunger away and blood sugar levels stable. Avoid all carbs, as they're most likely to be red zone or danger zone material.

For example:

- A sausage roll without the pastry shell, with a tub of plain unsweetened yoghurt, is better than a meat pie, which is better than a bag of hot chips.

- An egg and lettuce sandwich or ham and cheese sandwich with one slice of sourdough is better than the whole sandwich on ordinary bread. Or better still – if sandwiches are made to order, staff might be happy to make a small salad with egg, lettuce, ham and cheese, and these can usually be tackled without cutlery.

Snacking

Snacking can be helpful... or not

Snacking can help us moderate hunger between meals, tiding us over to the next one without sending our blood sugar high. But the wrong snacks, eaten the wrong way, easily undermine our efforts to reach a better weight.

Make snacking a conscious choice, rather than an absent-minded habit. First, have some water, then check – is this hunger? Or could it be one of my other food triggers? Does eating now fit with plans for my next meal?

If you still identify hunger, choose a snack that supports your weight goals: something **_high in protein and low in sugar_** (see some ideas in the box below).

It's not usually easy to find high-protein, low-sugar snacks at the office, or at nearby shops. So if you're not going to be home during the day, **_plan ahead for snacks_**.

Keep sight of the fact that it's not unhealthy to sometimes feel a little hungry and go without. We can just let it be.

Plan ahead for snacks

Plan **when** you'll snack, and **what** you'll have.

When

Decide on your meal and snack routine (Chapter 3 has more on regular eating). Regular snacks can be part of a healthy eating routine, especially if you've decided to eat five or six times per day. But if you aren't hungry when it's snack time, don't eat; it's probably a sign that your earlier meal was enough.

What

If you're going to be away from home during the day, pack food to take with you. Alternatively, if you're buying lunch at work, check the portion size, as it's likely to be larger than you need. Divide the portion into three parts, have two parts for lunch and save the remainder for a small meal or snack a few hours later.

The night-time snacker

Is this you? In front of the TV at 9 pm, winding down… reaching for something to put in your mouth. Food, alcohol, or both.

First – obviously you aren't alone (for me, it's chocolate). Evening snacking is very common. It's heavily associated with the reward of the relaxing wind-down, signalling an end to daytime cares and responsibilities. Because the context for night-time snacking (emotional release) is so closely connected to the snacking activity (a little food 'reward'), night-time snacking can be a strongly rooted habit.

There's also a deeper reason, though. We're biologically predisposed to seek fattening food (starchy carbs with added fat: danger zone food, in other words) at night, because **night-time carb-eating is a very effective way to store fat**. Fat storage is a priority for humans when food is scarce, but that's no longer a problem for most of us.

Evening snacking needn't be a habit for life. We can change it, like any other habit.

- **_Call it out_**. Stare it in the face and recognise night-time snacking for what it is. It's a habit, and even though it might be a biological preference, it doesn't seal your fate.

- **_Change the context_**. Do something different in the evening, for example:

  » Turn off the TV. Do something physical but low key, such as walking or yoga (high-intensity exercise too close to bedtime can interfere with sleep). Or get into a good book, learn a musical instrument, play cards or board games.

  » For TV nights, sit in a different chair or even move the TV to a different place. Changing the location of a habit is one way to break it – let this small difference trigger change.

- **_Tea ceremony_**. Have an 'end-of-eating' routine after your evening meal. Have a cup, pot or glass of your favourite non-sweetened, non-caffeinated, non-alcoholic drink. Then clean your teeth.

- **_No access_**. Avoid the means for snacking. Don't keep your snack trigger food in the house.

Ideas for supportive snacks

- A small handful of raw, unsalted nuts (about 20 nuts)

- Plain yoghurt (dairy) or plain cottage cheese

- A small can of tuna (preferably in water or olive oil; some of the flavoured varieties contain significant sugar)

- A boiled egg

- Canned or dry-roasted chickpeas

- A small portion of a high-protein, low-sugar left-over meal

- High-fibre green vegetables – celery sticks or raw broccoli florets are great. (Sounds weird, but try it! Completely different flavour and texture.) Have them on their own, or with home-made hummus or salsa dip.

Managing cravings

It's common to have food cravings, and usually not for a nice juicy capsicum or a bowl of tomatoes. (If you do crave those things, you may have a vitamin deficiency. Not joking.)

Cravings for high-carb, fatty, sugary or salty food are a big deal for many of us. Being controlled by cravings undermines our efforts to protect our bodies.

Try logic first

It's often possible to 'treat' a mild craving with awareness and logic. Remind yourself of your admiration for your body. Visualise what happens to your blood sugar and fat storage when you eat sugary food and acknowledge it takes you a step backwards from your goal.

Change the place and context, and use positive self-talk to support yourself as you move into a different activity.

Say it

Remember the language of empowerment back in Chapter 2? *'I don't…' (not 'I can't').*

Say it aloud and keep it casual: *'I just don't eat much sugar anymore, it doesn't agree with me.'* Verbalising the commitment helps make it real.

Resist the sales pitch

Advertisers spend billions of their clients' dollars every year trying to make us believe that food created out of highly processed carbs, with added fats and heavily flavoured with sugar or salt (often both), as well as artificial flavourings, is 'everyday food'. They tell us their products have a place in a healthy, balanced diet.

This is just not true. These products have no place in everyday eating. If you're yearning for packaged or fast food, remind yourself not to give advertisers the satisfaction! They don't have your best interests at heart – the stuff is dangerous. There's more about food advertising in Chapter 12.

Break it

Tackling the addiction head-on and going cold turkey on sugar and danger zone food is probably the best long-term way to manage cravings for danger zone food, but it's undeniably difficult. If you're up for the challenge, try some of these ideas.

Your body, your choice

Remember that you can eat it any time – *if you want to*. Nobody and nothing is stopping you. Sugar and danger zone food is easy to get hold of, and usually inexpensive. The only question is – at this exact moment you have already stopped eating it, so **do you really want to start again?**

Ride the wave

One of the best ways to manage a craving is to ride through it, with a high degree of awareness.

- Be aware that what you're experiencing is a craving. Know what triggers your cravings, and **expect** to feel it – watch for it, look out for it.

- When the craving hits, notice how it affects you, physically and mentally. Feel the sensation of desire building – are you salivating or fidgeting, your brain a jumble of incoherent wanting? (That's me anyway… yours might be similar, or not.)

- The sensation grows and feels all-powerful. But it's not all-powerful. Just like an ocean wave, after the peak has passed, the sensations fall away; they always do. You come out the other side, unharmed.

Eat more protein

Studies have shown that having frequent, higher protein meals may help to reduce filler food cravings.

Bitter might be better

Some research shows that eating bitter food may help prevent sugar cravings. There's also some evidence that bitter foods have a general appetite-suppressing effect. Try black coffee and green tea, rocket or radicchio leaves, brussels sprouts and kale.

Get enough sleep

Poor sleep is a powerful driver of sweet cravings. Chapter 8 has more on the connection between sleep, cravings and weight gain.

Withdrawal woes

Research shows that high-sugar food has all the hallmarks of an addictive substance, so be ready for real withdrawal symptoms. Symptoms vary, and how intensely you feel them will depend on how much sugar you're used to eating. You might feel anxious, depressed or irritable, find it difficult to concentrate or have increased sugar or carb cravings. It's also common to have physical symptoms like a headache and fatigue.

Increasing protein, fibre and water can help to reduce withdrawal symptoms. So can the knowledge that it doesn't last forever (generally only three to five days). And that you come out the other side already far healthier.

Don't substitute with artificial sweeteners – they won't help, and may make matters worse. Chapter 4 has more on sweeteners.

Mitigation

If you do 'give in' to a craving, don't beat yourself up about it! Get constructive instead. Be ready to experience a blood sugar dip and another sugar craving shortly afterwards, and work out how you'll respond to it.

A tablespoon of apple cider vinegar or psyllium husk (or both) in a full glass of water, will help slow the blood sugar impact a little.

Living with younger children

Parenthood is a fast-moving feast. Children change constantly and often unpredictably, so our routines often change too, bringing new challenges for establishing and keeping healthy eating habits, and instilling those habits in them, too.

Grandparents often play a large role in children's everyday lives, including mealtimes. If you're someone who has regular care of children (whether as a grandparent or otherwise), this section is equally for you.

Healthy eating habits are good for children too

The Five for Life habits are just as applicable to our children's eating as they are to our own. As children are inclined to do as we do, rather than do as we say, showing children healthy eating habits offers them the best likelihood of maintaining healthy weight for the rest of their lives.

Teach simple aspects of lifelong habits:

- Appreciating their own bodies
- Eating breakfast
- Drinking plenty of water
- Finishing eating before they're full
- Understanding how to recognise unhealthy carbs and the danger zone (carbs plus fat and sugar/salt) – and limiting them to rare occasions
- Never using food as a reward for 'good' behaviour
- Understanding that food advertising is clever and cynical, generated by a powerful industry that does not care about their health
- Eating carefully, with gratitude and attention, chewing slowly and thoroughly.

As children get older, we can add more detail and explain the reasons. Involve them in shopping and cooking the 'healthy habits' way.

Eating with children

Growing children need more food, more frequently, than we do. But when we're constantly preparing food or participating in meals, or both, it can be easy to lose sight of the fact that our nutritional needs are different. If we eat as our growing children do, then we will grow too – out, not up!

Carbs and quantities

Food that's good for children might not be good for us. Children do need more carbs than most adults do. High-quality carbs, of course – children shouldn't get used to regularly eating high-GI refined carbs, as it will set them up for health and weight problems later in life.

Growing children, particularly if they're active with sport, need larger servings of their evening meal than most of us, especially if we're minding our weight. Explain to children that your evening portion is very small because your body has stopped growing. It needs the night-time to finish digesting what you've already eaten during the day.

Leftovers – think differently about food wastage

Children's leftovers aren't somehow calorie-free. Eating what they leave is as much a waste as throwing it out, and moves us away from our ideal weight.

Save leftovers for another meal or snack, give safe scraps to pets, start a worm farm, compost at home, or use your local council organics collection. If your council doesn't have an organics collection system, agitate until they get one! Sending food waste to landfill causes significant greenhouse gas emissions. Meanwhile, see if a neighbour would like scraps for their pets or garden.

'Treats' and party food

Change the way you look at food treats

Buying 'treats' for children that are made of sugar (e.g. lollies or sweet drinks) or are in the danger zone (e.g. chips, cakes, biscuits, chocolate) puts them in harm's way, literally. Apart from the direct risk of gaining excess weight during childhood, regularly providing high-sugar and danger zone food sets up unsafe eating habits, burdening their future from an early age. Aggressive marketing of danger zone items, not only to children but to their parents and caregivers, is a major cause of rapidly increasing childhood obesity.

Children are observant! They notice, although probably not consciously, when we implicitly 'accept' food advertising by buying the shiny things. If we don't buy processed food treats, children won't be eating them (not at home, anyway) and they won't be in the house tempting us, either. Allow children's precious, growing bodies to develop in a way that will carry them safely through the rest of their lives.

Substitute

Help children learn that treats are normally non-food things, like fun outings and activities. Do something they enjoy together – play games, or take the dog out.

Encourage children to recognise real food treats like a colourful platter of fresh, crunchy vegetable sticks with cheese, nuts and fresh fruit. Home-made avocado dip, decorated boiled egg heads. In winter, thick lentil, pumpkin or tomato soup with wholegrain toast. Welcoming hungry children, just back from the park or school, with a plate of good food is a great way to condition them to look forward to it.

Parties

It's virtually impossible to avoid high-sugar and danger zone food at children's parties. There will be fizzy drinks, cupcakes, chips, lollies and chocolate.

Realistically – it's fine for children to understand that some types of foods are okay for parties, as long as they have just a little. Talk to them, explaining the idea of filler and danger zone food:

- That regularly eating this type of food now can make them sick as they get older

- That their growing bodies want real food, which has lots of nutrients

- That the best fun you have at parties isn't anything to do with the food

- That it's okay to have a little, on rare special occasions like parties, but it's not everyday food. And to be ready for their brain to demand more of it, and to know how to stop.

At the supermarket

It's incredibly wearing when children nag at the supermarket for 'treat' food. And they do – this is the point of food advertising. Advertisers would be out of work if they didn't successfully appeal to their targets.

The best solution, of course, is to shop without children, such as on the way home from work, or on the way to school pick-up, or when someone else is home to look after them. But that's often just not possible, and I've had plenty of supermarket horror trips.

A least-worst approach can be to have a 'lolly day' once a week. When my boys were school-age, it was Monday. If it wasn't Monday, there was no point asking. On Mondays, they could choose one item. Did it work all the time? Of course not! And no doubt my children ate more sweets than some children, and less than others.

The best of the bunch is chocolate, in my opinion. It generally has the least artificial colouring and flavouring, and a little of the good stuff (protein, calcium and some vitamins in the cocoa and milk). Contrast with jelly snakes – no calcium or other minerals, no vitamins, no protein. And a range of colours and flavourings to make them more attractive, because who really wants to swallow 10 teaspoons of plain sugar?

CHAPTER ELEVEN

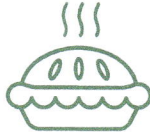

WHAT'S COOKING?

This bit isn't exciting and it's definitely not glamorous.

It's just the coal-face – everyday cooking and food shopping. But it's absolutely essential, and it's here that many of the healthy eating habits will be created, and unhealthy ones discarded.

So let's dive into the very practical side of things: planning meals, shopping and cooking. In this chapter, we'll talk about:

- *Meal planning and preparation* – this section is especially for people who usually don't have much time to spend in the kitchen. It looks at what to do when you get home late, some quick meal suggestions, and advice about some of the 'faster' options such as pre-made meals

- *Shopping* – maximise your chances that food-buying supports healthy habits.

Meal planning and preparation

A healthy approach to food and eating does mean spending time and headspace on food preparation. How much of a change this will be for you personally depends on what you're used to cooking, and how much of a role processed food or takeaway has played in your daily eating up until now.

Two things will help:

- *First* – remember there's no need to change everything at once. No need for a sudden and dramatic conversion, because this is the sort that's more likely to come unstuck later.

- *Second* – planning meals ahead makes life much easier. It saves time, but it also saves headspace. I'm know I'm not the only one whose stress levels shoot up when I hear *'What's for dinner, Mum?'*

The Five for Life approach means having the majority of our energy intake in the first part of the day, and leaving the last meal light. This might mean that on weekdays or workdays, the most practical solution is to eat a smaller portion of the evening meal, and save most of it for a more substantial meal at lunchtime the following day. On days when cooking and eating can be more relaxed, serve the main meal at lunchtime.

Greater acceptance of working from home has allowed more of us better flexibility around meal timing. If this is you, make the most of it.

Getting home late

Getting home at 6 pm or later is common after a day out, or a day at work. It can be a particularly stressful few hours, especially if you've picked up children from childcare or after-school sport or other activities. Everyone's tired, and often hungry too.

Assuming you're in bed by 10 pm, you need to *finish eating before 7 pm* to make the most of your overnight fat-burning fast. No point beating around the bush – this bit is difficult. It takes maximum forward planning and realistic expectations (on yourself, and by others).

- Rule no. 1 – Weeknight dinners are not gourmet events.

- Rule no. 2 – Takeaway bought on the way home is not the answer. It will almost certainly be a high-carb, high-sugar, high-fat affair. The 5–10 minutes it takes to order and collect is not much less than what it takes to make a simple meal at home.

- Rule no. 3 – All the other chores and demands can (almost always) wait until after dinner.

- Rule no. 4 – If you don't have an evening meal at all, it doesn't matter, but look after children who do need a meal.

Planning, cooking and food preparation

Getting a meal on the table within 30 minutes of walking in the door is not easy, but it's doable, and gets easier with practice.

Planning ahead is essential. Planning starts with your shopping list, then a basic weekday meal plan. Sometimes, of course, things change, and your plans might be out the door the moment you walk in. If that's the case, go for one of the very simple 10-minute meals, with staples you have on hand, like eggs, cheese and everyday vegetables, canned fish or pulses.

Pick three or four meals you can make in about 20 minutes without a recipe. Now and then, rotate a couple of things on your menu with something different. It makes shopping much easier, and reduces time and waste. Most importantly – it *reduces the amount of headspace you need to get dinner ready*.

Plenty of simple, nutritious meals can be on the table within half an hour. Share ideas with friends or go online when you run out of inspiration. An astounding array of creative, generous people have put together their own suggestions for the universally taxing 'What's for dinner?' question.

Quick meal ideas

Meal preparation time is often mostly attributable to the chopping-up bit. Minimise how much chopping is involved – frozen vegetables help a lot in this regard.

5-minute meals – the best workday meal is the one you made earlier!

- Leftovers from a previous meal, ready to re-heat and eat.
- A meal you prepared the previous day, or on the weekend.

10-minute meals

- Poached eggs on cooked spinach or mixed vegetables.
- Chickpeas with fried red capsicum, spring onion, kale and cherry tomatoes. Add bacon if you like, for a delicious smoky flavour.
- Fish fillets microwaved from frozen, on a bed of mixed vegetables with tomato passata (crushed tomatoes, in a can or jar). Sprinkle with cheese for more flavour, protein and calcium.
- Thinly sliced chicken fillets or prawns under the griller with a drizzle of olive oil and salt and pepper. Serve with steamed broccoli, green beans and peas. Add some interest to the veggies with home-made salad dressing.

20-minute meals

- Poached, BBQ, fried or grilled meat, poultry or fish with vegetables and salad. For people in the house who need carbs, add mashed root vegetables. A combination of potato, carrot and cauliflower is tasty, and lower in carbs and higher in nutrients than plain potato.
- Stir-fry a protein source with non-starchy vegetables. Fry in a little olive oil, and finish with a teaspoon of sesame oil, soy sauce and black pepper. Steer clear of purchased stir-fry sauces, as they're mostly high in sugar.

- Tuna mornay, using a large quantity of small-chopped vegetables (e.g. broccoli, spring onions, capsicum, celery, green beans). If you're feeding growing children who need the extra carbs, add cooked pasta to their serve.

Something you prepared earlier... batch cooking

Include in your menu-list meals that can be made in bulk and last well in the fridge, or can be frozen. I use mince-based things for this, including shepherd's pie, chilli con carne, bolognaise or meatballs, as well as slow-cooked curries and stews.

Poached chicken breasts are a great standby. Throw a couple in a saucepan on the weekend or if you have a minute through the week. Use them for lunch or dinnertime salads, or for an extremely quick stir-fry.

Not worth it – pasta sauces and other ready-made sauces

Ready-made sauces for adding to vegetables, chicken or other protein as 'simmer sauces' and meal bakes seem like a quick meal solution but these products will work against your health goals. They're heavily processed, containing added sugar, vegetable oil and artificial additives.

The only exception is plain passata – Italian-style cooked tomatoes packaged in glass jars. It's an excellent, versatile base for many meals.

Appendix C summarises principles for building simple meals. The Five for Life website has more ideas for quick meals.

Pre-made meals

Can pre-made meals have a place in healthy eating habits? It depends...

A wide range of frozen and fresh pre-made meals are available in supermarkets, and there's a growing industry in ready-made meals delivered to your door, either completely prepared, or in ready-to-cook kits.

Meal kits vary enormously in quality. Many of the meals are high in carbs, saturated fat and refined vegetable oil, although it's possible to find healthy choices. Be aware that this is an expensive way to eat. Food-delivery companies need to process the order, assemble, prepare and pack ingredients, and deliver them to our door. Those costs, plus a profit margin, are added to the ordinary cost of buying ingredients. And they all come with *a lot* of packaging.

The plus side is that meal kits and fully made meals remove the 'What's for dinner?' stress, and provide an interesting variety and ideas for your own cooking. Meal kits can also be a good way to help non-cooks in your family become more interested and involved in the process. And receiving only the ingredients you need for each meal, while an expensive way to do it, can result in less food wastage.

The main things to look out for are *adequate protein, added sugar, excessive or poor-quality carbs*, and *vegetable oil*. Check the ingredients list and nutrition panel carefully, and look for meals that are:

- high in protein from unprocessed sources (at least 20 g per 300-calorie serve)
- low in carbs (not more than 40 g per 300-calorie serve). This means avoiding meals with bread, pastry, rice, pasta and potatoes
- low in sugar (less than 5 g per serve)
- high in non-starchy vegetables, especially greens
- low-to-medium saturated fat (not more than 5 g per serve) and not made with vegetable oil unless it's cold-pressed olive, nut or coconut oil
- as little processed as possible.

As most meal kit serves are well over 300 calories, you'll need to do some rough maths to work out the protein, carb and fat content. If you choose something that only comes in larger serves, section out part to have for breakfast or lunch the next day.

Avoiding vegetable oil is particularly difficult in pre-made meals, as it's an inexpensive and therefore widely used source of fat. Check the ingredients list, and reject meals where vegetable oil is in the top five.

A warning – I've found <u>some</u>, but not many, pre-made meals that meet all the criteria. Generally, meals made up of vegetables or salad, dressed with olive oil and unsweetened vinegar or plain yoghurt, together with a whole protein source (e.g. a piece of fish, chicken or meat) are your best bets. Good-quality vegetarian meals may be more difficult to source. Limit how often you use pre-made meals.

Making sure children get what they need

No one should be eating large meals in the evening. But children are notorious for not eating what you packed them for school lunch, or for not making great choices if they're buying food at school. This means breakfast and dinner are important times to make sure they get enough protein and vegetables.

Children need higher amounts of high-quality carbs than adults, especially if they're active with sport. If they had sandwiches for lunch, and other carbs during the day (including sugary filler-food), the evening portion of carbs can be small. Put most of your emphasis on quality protein and vegetables, and help set them up for good eating habits later in life.

Quick-as-a-flash, high-quality carbs for kids

Prepare weekday carbs on the weekend or when you have time, and refrigerate or freeze them. They can be added to children's serves of any of the quick meal suggestions.

- Cook pasta and refrigerate it. Wholegrain is best, although it can take a while to get used to its nutty flavour and heavier texture. When reheating, stir through a tablespoon of pesto, or add a little butter, grated cheese and black pepper.

- Cook a mix of quinoa and wild rice or brown rice. This freezes well, reheating in the microwave in seconds.

- Sweet potato and carrot mash will keep in the fridge for two to three days.

- Bread has its place – but only some types. A slice of wholegrain, grilled with cheese or under a poached egg, is a good addition for a growing child. If your child isn't used to the flavour, keep offering it; their taste buds will eventually change. You're in charge of shopping, so buy stuff that counts.

What if it's just too late?

If it's late and there's not enough time to finish eating three hours before bed – ask yourself if you really need dinner tonight. Or do you just 'feel like it' because it's a strongly ingrained habit? Go back through your day and visualise everything you ate and drank (apart from water) laid out in front of you. *Does your body need more – and if so, more of what exactly?*

If it's too late but you're truly hungry, have a small handful of nuts, or a tub of plain yoghurt or cottage cheese, drink a cup of herbal tea, clean your teeth and go to bed.

The bottom line on meal prep

Preparing your own quick and nutritious meals is key to establishing good eating habits. If you're not used to cooking, or you're at work all day, it takes planning and practice to get the knack.

Instant, not Insta. Dinner doesn't have to be magazine-worthy. Go for simple, nutritious and light evening meals.

None is fine. You won't suffer if you miss dinner altogether, even if you haven't quite had your day's protein quota. Treat it as an opportunity to extend your overnight fast, burning even more fat between now and breakfast tomorrow morning.

Do feed the children. But meals need only be small and balanced – there's nothing wrong with eggs on wholegrain toast with carrots, broccoli and peas!

Call a friend. Everyone has a few life hacks for quick, easy meals; ask friends for their favourite standby.

Shopping

Most of what we eat, we will have bought ourselves. If we don't buy it, we won't eat it. Don't kid yourself that it's for visitors. (If it really is for visitors – do they deserve things that you wouldn't eat yourself?)

Food shopping is serious business. Make it work *for you*, not against you.

What, when, who and how

What

Make a shopping list and stick to it. One exception to the 'stick to it' rule is if your healthy staples (e.g. pulses, eggs, canned fish, raw nuts) are on special.

When

Be aware of your own trigger times, when you're more likely to buy food that's not helpful for you. This might be after work when you're tired, or when you're hungry. Avoid shopping at trigger times.

Who

Do whatever it takes to shop without the company of children. Children's power to influence food purchases is well known to supermarkets and food manufacturers, and they deliberately make the most of it. Most supermarket shelves are cynically stocked in a way that places items attractive to children at their eye-level, or at the checkout.

How

Before you enter the shop, take a moment. A deep breath. Now set your intention: to shop in the way that is kindest to you and your body. To stick with your list and not be distracted by food advertising (there's more about food advertising in Chapter 12).

Recognise your own trigger foods, and where they're likely to be stocked. Relax – these things don't control you, and nor do the advertisers trying to make you put them in your trolley. Use your intention and your list, to just walk on by. If you need to, use the 'ride the wave' technique described in Chapter 10 to manage cravings.

Sometimes you hear advice to 'shop in the outside aisles'. I have no idea how that was dreamed up, and it's not good advice. Perfectly healthy food staples are often somewhere in the middle of a shop (e.g. canned vegetables and fish, nuts and loose dried pulses and whole grains). Not to mention pet food, household items, condiments, long-life and alternative milks, and tea and coffee.

Read food labels for all packaged food. If sugar is one of the top four ingredients, or is more than 10 g per 100 g, *leave it on the shelf*. An exception to that rule is for condiments like sauces and chutneys, that we use only in small amounts for flavour.

Consider online shopping

Online shopping can be a great way to save time and money, and not be distracted by children and 'special deals' on red zone carbs or danger zone food.

Shopping lists

Shopping lists are vital for sticking to healthy eating habits. They also save money and help reduce food wastage.

Shopping lists

I keep the list on the kitchen bench, and add to it during the week when I remember things. It starts with the 'every week' items, followed by pantry staples running low, plus extras if we plan to see friends over the weekend.

- ✓ Eggs
- ✓ Nuts (raw, mixed)
- ✓ Milk
- ✓ Block of cheddar cheese
- ✓ Meat – generally kangaroo mince or steak, chicken fillets, fresh or frozen fish
- ✓ Dog food
- ✓ Vegetables – these vary depending on the season and what I'm planning to cook, but staples are kale, spring onions, capsicum, broccoli, sweet potato, salad leaves, cucumber, tomatoes, carrots, cauliflower, eggplant, Asian greens, celery, green beans
- ✓ Passata (jars or cans of tomato puree). Avoid pre-made pasta sauces and other simmer sauces; they're generally heavy in sugar and other additives
- ✓ Coconut cream
- ✓ Canned chickpeas, kidney beans and black beans, loose uncooked lentils
- ✓ Quinoa and wild rice
- ✓ Pasta (for my two growing sons)
- ✓ Rolled oats, muesli or Vita Brits (ditto)
- ✓ Canned fish (plain, in olive oil or spring water)
- ✓ Frozen vegetables – to replace things used up over the week
- ✓ Stone-ground spelt and wheat sourdough bread from our local bakery.

Plan for five main meals

Before leaving for the shops, finesse the list: decide what you'll be cooking for at least five main meals, with enough for leftovers. Let these meals be simple, easy-to-prepare things.

Vegetables

Fresh, frozen or canned? All are fine, and useful for different purposes.

Fresh

Most vegetables do taste better fresh, and of course are essential for salads and raw vegetable dishes. There are lots of extra bits, leaves and ends, so if you're a keen cook, or have chooks or like to home-compost, there's plenty for everyone.

When in season, fresh veg are inexpensive, tasty and full of nutrients. If you can buy from a growers' market, you'll be directly supporting local farmers and helping to reduce your carbon footprint.

Frozen

Frozen vegetables are generally cheaper than fresh, unless it's the peak of the season. They're also frequently higher in nutrients (apart from in-season, locally grown produce), as they're typically picked when perfectly ripe and washed, blanched (in boiling water – no chemicals), and frozen and packaged within a few hours of harvest.

Other benefits are that they:

- leave no wastage – no peelings, ends and outer leaves
- are an excellent way to get fiddly veg such as peas, sweet corn kernels, broad beans and edamame (soy) beans
- offer a good mixture in small quantities – especially good for singles or couples
- are great for a quick meal when you get home late (no chopping-up!).

Buy Australian to support our own food producers, and minimise the carbon burden of food.

Canned

Canned vegetables are a useful pantry standby, but there are some things to watch out for.

Tomatoes. There is potential for bisphenol-A (BPA) in the lining of cans to leach into tomatoes due to their high acid content, and this is more likely to happen if cans are damaged or dented. Manufacturers have moved away from BPA, but replacement liners are chemically similar and may still be implicated in health risks including childhood obesity. Food Standards Australia and similar bodies in the US and Europe report no scientific evidence of health risks of BPA at the quantities we would ingest through eating canned food... but if you can reduce or avoid it, why not? A good alternative to canned tomatoes that works in most contexts is passata – Italian-style cooked tomatoes in glass jars. Essentially the same as cans, but a smoother consistency.

Pulses. Most pulses can be bought already cooked and canned, which is definitely convenient. On the other hand, home-cooked pulses can be frozen in small batches for use later so it's a time-saver in the long-run to cook your own. However, I'm probably not the only one who's full of good intentions for pre-cooking my pulses, but in reality end up mainly relying on cans.

Pulses aren't acidic, so there's much lower risk of BPA leaching.

Other canned vegetables. Plenty of other vegetables (and fruit) come in cans too – e.g. sweet corn, mushrooms, asparagus and beetroot. Highly acidic items, such as pineapple and pickled beetroot, do risk BPA leaching.

Canned vegetables are heated to high temperatures to kill micro-organisms before sealing, and this leaves most of them tasting quite different from fresh or frozen products. Canned fruit is steeped in either fruit syrup or fruit juice; either way, a high-sugar item.

Beware the supermarket trap – go shopping with your eyes open

The purpose of a supermarket is to sell us food. In particular, supermarkets would like us to buy food that carries the highest profit margin for them. Supermarkets pursue profit by arranging the food they want us to buy in the most visible places, and by using pricing techniques to try to make us buy more of it.

Predictably, the packaged food that has the highest profit margin for manufacturers and supermarkets (even when it's on 'special') is the food that is cheapest to produce. Cheap-to-produce food is frequently made of low-quality carbs and added sugar, with low nutritional value.

The food most likely to be on special, and at the biggest discount, will be red zone and danger zone food – high-sugar breakfast cereal, ice cream, chips, chocolate and lollies. A recent Australian study of price promotions in supermarkets found that these junk food items were on special *almost twice as often* as staples such as canned pulses, bread and frozen vegetables. The danger zone food was also offered at much higher discounts than the staples.[59]

On top of this, producers of junk food frequently pay supermarkets for premium display locations: they pay to have their products in the most tempting places, such as ends-of-aisles, and at checkouts. They also pay incentives for other forms of promotions, including multi-buy pricing and discount specials. If it's cheap, remember that someone always pays the price. Is it you, or your health? Is it the farmers or factory workers? The environment?

Chapter 12 has more about food advertising, and how to protect ourselves from it.

---

[59] Riesenberg (2019) Price promotions by food category and product healthiness in an Australian supermarket chain.

The bottom line on shopping

Go alone. Leave children and other helpers at home if possible.

Don't go hungry. Shop at a time when you won't be triggered by hunger or anxiety.

Take a list. Stick to it.

Be alert. Know that the food that's most likely to catch your eye (and especially your child's eye) in the supermarket won't be the healthiest. It's been placed there for a reason. Protecting your health is not a driving motivator for either supermarkets or food manufacturers.

Read the fine print. Always check labels before buying packaged food. Chapter 12 has more on what to look for on food labels.

CHAPTER TWELVE

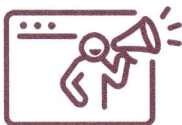

FOOD ADVERTISING – DON'T BUY IT

Food advertising has a lot to answer for in terms of the global epidemic of overweight and obesity.

Aggressive marketing of highly processed food, particularly in the danger zone (carbs plus fat and sugar or salt), has generated an insidious illusion that danger zone food is a 'normal' part of life, and it's almost impossible to shift.

Don't underestimate the power of advertising. In the face of well-funded, constant insistence that we should expect to eat danger zone food as part of our everyday life, establishing and keeping healthy eating habits has never been more difficult.

But forewarned is fore-armed, so this chapter exposes some of the *traps and tricks of food advertisers.*

In this chapter, we'll talk about:

- *Food advertising versus food labelling* – the point of food advertising, and how to avoid being sucked in (use product labels)

- *Advertising tricks and traps* – recognising them, and pushing back against manipulation
- *Myths and magic words* food advertisers use, and what they really mean.

Food advertising vs. food labelling

Food manufacturers dedicate serious money to making you want to buy

Food and beverage manufacturers spend an enormous amount of money advertising their products. Up-to-date figures for Australia aren't readily available, but in 2016, advertising in the 'food, produce and dairy' category was nearly $400 million. This doesn't include what advertisers spend on incentives to encourage supermarkets to discount and promote their products.[60]

All food products being advertised are processed and manufactured

When was the last time you saw whole, unprocessed food being advertised on TV or bus shelters, or in magazines? Nobody advertises oranges, chicken fillets, or chickpeas, except as a supermarket special. And even that has a cynical motive – supermarkets advertise staples on special as 'loss leaders', to encourage us to do our shopping with them rather than elsewhere.

The point of advertising manufactured food is to make us want to buy more of it, not to make us healthier. Food advertisers are interested in healthy profits, not healthy people.

---

[60] And it doesn't include advertising by fast-food outlets either. For example, fast-food advertising in the US in 2019 was $5 billion (USD). A similar per capita spend in Australia would be around $700 million (AUD).

Food labels aren't advertising – use them

The only piece of food packaging that isn't advertising is the part that the government forces food manufacturers to include – the *ingredients list and the nutrition information panel*.

Food manufacturers hate the nutrition panel and fought for many years to prevent it becoming law.[61] It was introduced in Australia in 2003, and the industry still fights it – in particular, opposing changes to increase information about sugar content. Industry excuses are mainly that a change would be 'costly'; apparently, among other things, they would need to educate staff and get legal advice, and manage increased calls to their customer help lines. Not to mention needing to update their packaging! Imagine the printing expenses. Interesting to know that mandatory 'added sugar' requirements were added to food labelling laws in the US from January 2020, after a four-year phase-in period.

The nutrition panel is always tiny, and often in a place that's difficult to see. It's certainly not up the front, advertising the benefits of the product!

Food advertising often tells us what's *not* in the product – not what is in it. You know what I mean – the item is 'low fat', 'fat free', 'gluten-free' or has 'no added sugar'. But what *is* in the product? If you didn't make it yourself from scratch, you need to *get used to reading food labels*.

What to look for

Food labels aren't always easy to read. You need to know what to look for, without getting bogged down.

On the nutrition information panel, mostly look out for carbs: total carb content, and how much of that is sugar. Also check for total fat, trans fats and sodium, and keep these low.

---

[61] The nutrition information panel requirement was introduced in Australia in 2003. The food industry still resists attempts to increase food labelling, mostly opposing quantification of 'added sugars' and advisory labels for foods high in added sugars.

In the ingredients list, check for sugar and vegetable oil. Also look for artificial ingredients and additives such as preservatives, emulsifiers, artificial colourings and flavourings. Avoid them, or if you can't, compare products to find one that has these things low on the list.

'Sugar' on the label – what does it mean?

There are two types of sugars in food:

* *naturally occurring sugars,* like fructose in whole fruit, or lactose in milk (sometimes called 'intrinsic' sugars)

* *added sugars* (also called 'free' sugars). These include cane sugar, as well as sweeteners like honey or fruit juice concentrate, which are often used in manufactured food to give it a false, 'healthy-by-association' glow.

The nutrition panel doesn't have to identify whether sugar is naturally occurring in the food, or has been added.

Dissecting it

The nutrition panel at right is from a pack of untoasted muesli.

What should we be noticing?

* *Carbs.* 25.6 g carbs per serve. A serve is 45 g, which for this cereal is ½ cup; it's quite heavy due to the rolled oats. It has just under 60% carbs by weight, which is to be expected for a carb-based food.

* *Sugar.* 6.7 g per serve, or 15% sugar by weight. Not great, but just sneaks into an acceptable upper limit for sugar. Sugar forms part of the total carb content.

* *Type of sugar.* From the ingredients list, we see no 'added' sugar. The sugar will be naturally occurring from the fruit pieces, coconut and malt extract, and a little in the oats themselves.

* *Protein.* At just under 11% protein by weight, or just under 5 g per serve, this doesn't count as a significant source of protein.

The **serving size is 45g.** Each figure in the 'per serve' column is therefore the amount per 45 g.

Use the 'per serve' column to find out how much you'll consume if you eat the manufacturer's serving size.

Use the 'per 100 g' column to work out whether the food is, overall, a healthy choice (look for low sugar, with higher protein and fat). Use this column to compare food items.

Ingredients are listed from highest to lowest quantity. Look out for:

(1) Sugar under any name (e.g., fructose, maltose, maple syrup, fruit juice concentrate, or sucrose). This cereal doesn't list 'sugar', which means the sugar content is naturally occurring mainly from the dried fruit.

(2) Fats. Avoid products with 'vegetable oil' high on the list. In this cereal, fat comes mainly from the almonds, wheat bran and coconut, which are healthy sources.

(3) Things you *don't recognise.* The less recognisable the ingredients, the more the food has been processed.

Nutrition information
Breakfast cereal – untoasted muesli

Serving size – 45g

	Per serve	Per 100g
Energy	690kJ	1530kJ
Protein	4.9g	10.9g
Fat		
Total	3.6g	7.9g
Saturated	0.8g	1.8g
Carbohydrate		
Total	25.6g	56.9g
Sugars	6.7g	15g
Fibre	4.6g	10.3g
Sodium	7mg	15mg

Ingredients: Wholegrain Rolled Oats (70%), Dried Fruits, Wheat Bran, Almonds (1%), Coconut, Malt Extract (Barley), Vitamin E (Soy), Emulsifier (471)

Energy is shown in kilojoules (kJ). To convert to calories, divide by 4.2. This cereal has 164 calories per serve.

Protein. Food with at least 10 g per serve can claim to be a 'good source' of protein.

Fat is shown both as total fat, and saturated fat. Manufacturers also show other types of fat as a selling point (e.g. low trans fats, or high Omega 3). Check the ingredients list to find out the source of fat.

Carbs are shown both as total carbs (i.e., both starch and sugar), and how much of that is sugar. The information panel doesn't state how much is added sugar. Check the ingredients list to help work it out. Look for **sugar** content that is less than 10 g per serve *and* less than 15 g per 100 g. This cereal only just scrapes in.

Fibre doesn't have to be shown, but products that are high in fibre usually do. Bread or cereal should have at least 3 g per serve.

Sodium should be less than 120 mg per 100g, but up to 400 mg per 100 g is okay.

- *Fat.* About 8 g fat per 100 g. The ingredients list tells us this fat is from the almonds and coconut, which are both excellent sources of natural fats.

- *Fibre.* 4.6 g per serve (and about 10% by weight), which is quite good. Rolled oats are high in a valuable type of fibre, helping feed our 'good' gut biota.

How does this particular food rate?

Based on the ingredients list, and figures for carbs and sugar, protein and fat, it's pretty good as far as pre-made cereals go.

With around 26 g carbs per 45 g serve, it won't raise blood sugar too high. As most of the carbs are from wholegrain oats, the rise in blood sugar will be fairly slow, which is a good thing. Adding high-protein yoghurt and nuts would slow down the rise in blood sugar even more.

This product doesn't contain enough protein to make a proper meal, but a smaller serve (around 30 g) with a large dollop of plain yoghurt and a few more nuts or seeds, would be a healthy and substantial snack.

General guide for judging packaged food

- *Serving size.* Notice how big the serving size is, especially if it's a filler or danger zone food. Don't be surprised if a small bag of chips is 'two serves' per pack.

- *Energy.* Don't worry too much about energy value, but do make a mental note. A food that is high in energy for its weight, or per serving size, provides a significant part of our body's fuel needs. Do you really need it? Is it high-quality fuel?

- *Carbs.* Take a good look at carb content. If more than half the energy value comes from carbs, it's a carb-based food. Consider where this will fit in your overall carb intake for the day. While eating high-quality carbs is fine in the right quantities at the right time of day, remember that **carbs in processed food are seldom high quality, and therefore not helping you.**

- **Sugars.** Sugars are shown as a component of total carbs. If there's more than 10 g sugar per serve, or more than 15 g per 100 g, it's too much, and the item probably falls into the red zone carb category.

- **Fat.** The most important thing about fat is its source. A product high in natural, unprocessed fat, such as nuts or olive oil, isn't necessarily a problem. The problem lies mainly in processed vegetable oils and trans fats. Check the ingredients list for 'vegetable oil' or 'vegetable fat' and try to avoid it.

Tricks and traps

Food advertisers will use a wide range of 'healthy sounding' words to try to distract us from asking *How much sugar?*'

Fat free/low fat

In Australia, products can claim to be 'fat free' if they have no more than 0.15 g of fat per 100 g of product. 'Low fat' products must have no more than 3 g per 100 g.

So is fat free or low fat a good thing anyway? Not necessarily (jelly snakes are low fat, for example). We know three important things about fat:

1. Fat doesn't 'make you fat'. Dietary fat alone is not a significant contributor to excess weight.

2. Fat is only one of the three main components of all food, apart from water. If there's less fat, then there must be either more protein, more carbs (fibre, starch or sugar), or simply more water. Read the label to find out which it is.

3. The real problem is *heavily processed* fats (such as most vegetable oils except cold-pressed oils), and fat when it's presented in the danger zone formula: mixed with poor-quality carbs, plus sugar, salt or both.

Foods commonly marketed as 'low fat' and healthy include flavoured yoghurt, popcorn and muesli bars. These are likely to be high in carbs, including added sugars, and *they aren't healthy*.

Popcorn

'Buttered' or 'butter flavoured' popcorn contains heavily processed vegetable oils (not butter!), and is not a good choice.

Air-popped popcorn is low fat, but made up almost entirely of carbs. Popcorn is rapidly processed by our body into fuel, and unless we're about to go for a run, most of that energy will be stored as fat. And for some reason, popcorn always seems to come in enormous serves. Even the 'small' boxes.

Gluten-free

Gluten is a form of protein found in wheat grain, as well as some other grains. 'Gluten-free' food is simply missing this particular type of protein. It still contains fat, carbs (or both), and may contain some other form of protein.

Rice, potato, tapioca and maize (corn) are the most common wheat-flour replacements in gluten-free food. These types of flour, and the products they're made with, often have *more refined carbs, and less fibre*, than food made with gluten flour.

People with coeliac disease need to avoid all gluten, as it triggers an immune response that damages the gut. The rest of us can make whatever choices we like about eating gluten or not, but it's unlikely to have any bearing on our body fat composition – in spite of what food manufacturers would have us believe.

Gluten-free food is big business, as the supposed health claims have extended beyond coeliac sufferers into the general public. As with many trends, profit is often the motive, and there's little evidence to support gluten-free diets as a weight-management tool. In fact, studies show that when a person with gluten sensitivity or coeliac disease goes on a gluten-free diet, their weight often increases, possibly because their body absorbs more nutrients once gluten is excluded. Other reasons for weight gain on a gluten-free diet include the typically low fibre levels of gluten-free flour, which are often used to replace refined wheat flour. Some studies have also shown a gluten-free diet to reduce the gut biota associated with leanness.

Always check the nutrition panel. If the gluten-free product is bread, cake, pastry or biscuits, it still contains refined carbs, and these aren't healthful or helpful when your goal is weight reduction. A better approach to a gluten-free diet is to omit refined-grain products altogether.

No added sugar/no cane sugar

No added sugar

In Australia, food can claim it has no added sugar if it contains no added table sugar, sucrose, glucose, syrups or a range of other types of sugar, and no added honey, malt or fruit juice concentrate.

While it's useful to keep your eye out for 'no added sugar' in packaged food, it doesn't mean the food is low in sugars or carbs generally. A good example is fruit bread, averaging about 17% sugar by weight. Although most of this is from the fruit content, it still makes fruit bread a high-sugar offering. Check the nutrition panel to decide whether you'll buy it, and if so, how much to eat.

No cane sugar

The claim 'no cane sugar' simply means the food doesn't contain sucrose from sugar cane. Common substitutes include things that food manufacturers claim are healthy, such as honey, dates, fruit juice concentrate (often made from grapes) and coconut sugar.

All of these sugars just add empty carbs to our daily load. Check the label to see how many grams of sugar per 100 g before deciding if it's a safe choice.

High fibre

Foods high in fibre are, in general terms, good for our gut. They help move food through our digestive system, and feed the good bacteria that live there.

But high fibre doesn't always mean 'healthy'. Check the label to find out how much carbohydrate is in the high-fibre product – and how much of that is sugar. Sugared peanuts, for example, are high in fibre, but also high in carbs.

Enriched flour

'Enriched'… it sounds so good! When the term is used on food ingredient labels, it means something has been added to the food.

The term is usually used to refer to refined wheat flour that's been 'enriched' by replacing some micronutrients (normally B vitamins and iron) that were removed along with the natural fats and fibres during processing. Why are these removed in the first place? To give products a smoother texture and, importantly from the manufacturer's point of view, a much longer shelf-life.

Avoid products made with 'enriched' flour; it means the product is highly processed, with the grains entirely stripped of their natural goodness.

Low calorie

Under Australian food standards laws, packaged food can claim to be 'low calorie' if it contains less than 40 calories per 100 g. It can be 'reduced' calorie if it has 25% less energy than the comparison version of the food.

Packaged food that claims to be a low-calorie version generally has achieved this by removing fat, as fat is higher in calories per gram than either carbs or protein. The removed fat is usually replaced with carbs (including sometimes fibre), because they're cheaper than protein.

While total calories do matter, what matters more is the *source* of calories – if most calories in a piece of food are from sugar, starch, or highly processed vegetable oils, we're doing our body a serious disservice. A 100-calorie tin of fish or a couple of eggs are far kinder to our body than the same number of calories in cake.

High protein

High-protein packaged food can be helpful as a time-saver, *if* it's also low in processed vegetable fats and sugar. Watch out for highly processed items, though, with artificial additives.

If the food is made with mostly unprocessed ingredients and is low in sugar, with no artificial sweeteners, it might be a good choice. For instance, some muesli bars made with whole rolled oats, nuts and seeds, extra fibre and even added soy or whey protein, can be reasonable occasional snack options.

Low carb

Under Australian food labelling laws, a food claiming to be 'low carb' must contain at least 25% less carbohydrate than the same amount of the 'standard' version of the food.

Things to check:

- For the quantity you're going to eat, is the low-carb food going to make a significant difference?

- What has been put in to replace the carbs that are taken out? The food might be higher in protein, in fat, in indigestible fibre, or in moisture content. If it's fat, make sure it's not vegetable oil.

- Most importantly – how heavily processed is it, and what additives are included? The more processed food is, the worse it is for us, including our gut biota and our ability to maintain a healthy weight. Especially look out for non-sugar sweeteners – they're not a good thing. There's more about processed food in Chapter 4.

All natural

Great! 'All natural' might mean that the food is free from refined ingredients – but it might not mean that at all, because the term 'all natural' isn't regulated under Australian food standards. Our consumer protection laws mean that a manufacturer can't make false and misleading claims, but this is open to interpretation, especially when used in food advertising.

As for what impact 'natural' packaged food might have on your weight – most likely none, as this label on its own means nothing. What you're looking for is food that's natural *and unprocessed*.

The 'Health Star Rating'

The Health Star Rating system was introduced by the Australian government in 2014. The idea was that it would help people make healthy food choices when buying packaged food.

It's a voluntary system, so manufacturers choose whether they want to include a 'health star' rating on their label. It's also quite easy to manipulate, due to the system used to rate foods. The result is that foods high in sugar can gain a high rating if they are also high in protein, fibre or vitamins. For example, some popular breakfast cereals high in added sugar carry a 4-star rating because they have been fortified with extra protein and vitamins.[62]

My advice is to ignore the star rating on processed or packaged foods. Use the nutrition label and ingredients list to find out if the food is a healthy choice.

Organic

Organic food is grown without the use of synthetic chemicals (fertilisers, pesticides or herbicides). This method of food production is usually much better for soil health and the environment generally – so do choose organically grown food if it's available, and if you can afford it.

A good place to start is to buy organic food that doesn't have too much of a price differential – such as organic milk. You'll be supporting organic farmers as well as supporting soil health, insects and bees, and helping build demand for organic produce. Building demand will bring the price down over time so hopefully one day, organic production will be more common than other farming methods.

---

[62] The consumer advocacy group CHOICE has advocated a change in the algorithm used to rate foods, to penalise those with added sugar, but has been so far unsuccessful.

In terms of nutrition, organic meat and milk have been shown to contain much higher concentrations of valuable Omega-3 fatty acids, but there's no evidence that other organic food is necessarily higher in nutrients.

Choosing organic food helps reduce your exposure to 'environmental obesogens' – toxins in the environment that we suspect cause or contribute to the development of obesity by disrupting our endocrine system. Environmental obesogens include many pesticides, herbicides and other chemicals used in food production. They're also found in everyday products like household appliances and cleaners, detergents and even shampoos and cosmetics.

Free range

Buy free range whenever you can. Animals bred and pastured free range not only have a far better life, but have higher levels of healthy Omega-3 fat in their flesh, milk and eggs.

Sourdough

Sourdough refers to the way bread is made. Instead of yeast, a fermented starter culture is used to make the bread rise. Sourdough often, but not always, has a lower glycaemic index than bread made with yeast, meaning it will raise blood sugar more slowly (good for our weight). Sourdough contains higher levels of vitamins and minerals, and the fermentation process allows us to more easily absorb these nutrients.

Being a fermented food, good-quality, high-fibre sourdough helps our gut microbiome, which is also a good thing. Chapter 7 has more on the gut microbiome, and its role in overweight and obesity.

Sourdough has around the same total carbs as an equivalent serve of ordinary bread, so pay attention to how much you have.

High-protein cereal

Some cereals do have more protein than others, either naturally (as in plain rolled oats), or because they've been fortified. Two of the highest protein processed cereals on the market (Kellogg's® Nutri-Grain® and Weet-Bix™ Protein) are fortified with extra wheat and/or pea protein.

In Australia, food can claim to be a 'good source' of protein if it has at least 10 g per serve. Neither Weet-Bix™ Protein nor Nutri-Grain® quite makes it, at 9.4 g and 8.7 g per serve respectively. *And* both cereals are high in sugar – 7.3 g per serve for Weet-Bix™ Protein, and 9.6 g for Nutri-Grain®.

The bottom line is that *cereal is simply not 'high protein'*. If the nutrition panel shows that it really is high in protein (more than 20 g per 100 g), check the carb and sugar content too.

Keep a record of your favourites!

Seen any dodgy or laughable food advertising claims? Research them and enjoy de-coding the underlying message, and working out why the advertiser is using this particular message to sell the product.

Myths

There are plenty of food myths out there. As research continues to coalesce around agreement on the main components of a healthy diet, food manufacturers will work harder and harder to attempt to convince us that their product fits recommendations about healthy eating.

Remember how 'low fat' morphed into 'high sugar'? Fat content in many foods, for example, wonderfully healthy food like plain yoghurt, was replaced with low fat, sweetened 'fruit' and 'vanilla' versions to make this nutritious food more palatable and ultimately *unhealthy*.

We now know that overweight is primarily caused by sugar and highly processed foods, not natural fats (more about this in Chapter 4). So that debunks the first myth – 'low fat equals healthy'.

The second, insidious, myth we're sold is that it's perfectly fine to have danger zone food as part of an everyday diet. This myth was invented by the food industry, which vigorously promotes it.

'...can be enjoyed as part of a balanced diet'

For confectionery, the 'fine everyday' myth could also be called the 'treatwise trick'.

Be treatwise®' is an internationally used advertising tactic developed by the confectionery industry in a (mostly successful) bid to avoid government regulation of sugar advertising. It's a logo on the front of confectionery packs, which according to the industry is designed to:

> *'provide consumers with information to help explain the place that confectionery has, as a treat food, that can be enjoyed as part of a balanced diet and active lifestyle. [...] With its logo and tagline 'Enjoy a balanced diet',* Be treatwise® *helps consumers to understand the importance of eating treats in moderation.'*[63]

See what they did just there? Intentional or not, these words seem to be sending the wrong sort of messages.

- *It's a 'treat'.* Sugar, an addictive-like substance of no nutritional benefit, which substitutes for nutritious food choices (in your appetite and your wallet), is a special reward, a source of joy or delight. *What?*

- *It's something you 'enjoy'.* You're entitled to be happy, and you can *only really be happy if you eat sugar.* Especially if your friends are eating sugar too.

---

[63] https://www.betreatwise.info/about-be-treatwise/#.

- *It can be part of a 'balanced' diet.* If you find yourself addicted, and eat more than a 'serve', or in substitution for, or on top of, real, nutritious food, you're *greedy with no self-control.*

- *It's fine as long as you couple it with an 'active lifestyle'.* If you don't go the gym and work it all off, *you're just lazy.*

Processed items with high added sugar are **simply not part of a healthy, balanced diet.**

'Discretionary' foods

The Australian Dietary Guidelines describe certain foods as 'discretionary', advising that they 'can be included sometimes *in small amounts* by those who are *physically active*, but are not a necessary part of the diet' [my emphasis].[64]

'Discretionary food' as described in the Guidelines is poor in nutrients and high in calories. In Five for Life, it's red zone carbs, and/or danger zone food, and it includes:

- cakes and biscuits
- confectionery (including ice cream and gelato) and chocolate
- pastries and pies
- processed meats and fattier/salty sausages
- potato chips and crisps, and other fatty or salty snack foods
- sugar-sweetened soft drinks and cordials, sports and energy drinks and alcoholic drinks.

The Guidelines also include butter, cream, and spreads containing mostly saturated fats as discretionary foods. Strictly speaking, saturated fat isn't necessary in our diet, because our body can make its own, but I don't view butter and cream in the same category as the other things on this list. They are produced with minimal processing, and while they're not a necessary part of our diet, they are fine in small quantities. Chapter 4 has more detail on saturated fats.

---

[64]   National Health and Medical Research Council (2013) *Australian Dietary Guidelines.* Canberra: NHMRC https://www.nhmrc.gov.au/adg.

In terms of *how often* we can have discretionary food, the Guidelines don't give much indication. What they do say is that to keep up with our generally over-fed state, most of us would need to be doing moderate-intensity exercise *for at least 45–60 minutes every day* to avoid piling on extra body fat. As they point out:

> 'There is limited capacity for including energy-dense discretionary foods in nutritious dietary patterns within the energy requirements of many Australians.'

In short – if you aren't doing around 60 minutes of serious exercise every day, you can't afford to be eating much *(if any)* of this stuff. For most of us, that means taking special care to avoid these foods, especially while we're still moving towards our ideal weight.

'Happiness' in the danger zone?

Food advertisers would have us believe that eating discretionary foods will make us happy. We know this isn't true. But sugary, danger zone foods do feel good at the moment we put them in our mouth. That's the point, and it's why food manufacturers make this type of product. It's also why we make cakes and desserts for special occasions with family and friends.

Danger zone food fuels overeating – there are no two ways about it. Recent research details the way that carbs interact with fat (e.g. cake) to greatly increase our perception of reward. When we're faced with high-carb, high-fat food, we have a much greater 'willingness to pay' – we're intensely attracted to it. We're also more likely to underestimate the number of calories in food made of refined carbs combined with fat, especially with extra sugar.[65] For most people, the carbs plus fat and salt formula seems to have the same effect – for example, salted chips and crisps.

Recognise the addictive effect of the danger zone foods, and recognise the manufacturers' intent – they're very keen for us to keep buying the stuff.

---

[65] DiFeliceantonio (2018) Supra-additive effects of combining fat and carbohydrate on food reward.

Take a deep breath. You love your body, respect and admire it, and want to keep it safe from harm.

What, never?

Nobody is preventing you from eating whatever you like; it's always your own choice. If you decide to buy a 'discretionary' product, do it consciously, and resist 'buying' the advertising message. Be clear about why you're choosing the product, and what place it has in your overall food choices. Make it a rare occasion, and be mindful of its addictive potential.

If you're managing well at your happy weight, confectionery or danger zone food can safely be a now-and-then (monthly or perhaps weekly) event, in small serves. If you're struggling with sugar addiction or are above your target weight, do your best to just say no. If cold turkey is too painful or backfires into a negative 'deprivation' mindset, a good choice is a small piece of plain dark chocolate (minimum 75% cocoa). The higher the cocoa content, generally the lower the sugar, but do check the label.

Once you're physically and mentally where you want to be, re-assess the frequency with which you have discretionary foods. You might decide to stick with mostly leaving them out of your life. Remember, you're not imagining it – danger zone food has real, addictive-like properties, and needs to be treated with caution.

CHAPTER THIRTEEN

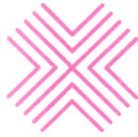

THAT'S ALL FOR NOW

I hope that after reading *Five for Life*, you're feeling confident and equipped with an approach to healthy eating that's easy to remember and put into practice.

The message I really want you to take to heart is that healthy eating is not just about what we eat, and any eating plan that's based on that idea is bound to fail. Healthy eating is about mindset (self-care, and the *why* of eating), timing (*when* we eat), diet (*what* we eat and *what* we drink), and action (*how* we eat).

In a nutshell

It's a long book… I know! So here's a recap of what it's all about, a quick reminder you can check back on as you make your own way towards your happy weight and a healthier future.

Part I sets out the Five Habits that form the why, when, what and how of eating:

1. *Treasure your body*. Keep your own body's welfare a priority and show kindness and compassion for yourself. Don't 'go on a diet' – no severe calorie restriction or cutting out food groups. Manage stress. Prioritise sleep. If you work shifts, know that you

need even more planning than most people to protect yourself. Check out the tips on stress, sleep and shift working in Chapter 8. And if you're going through pregnancy or menopause, Chapter 9 has more on how to care for your weight.

2. ***Eat at the right time***. Eat when you're hungry (and not when you're not). Learn to recognise your own hunger signals, and modify portion sizes to help your stomach sense when it's had enough. Eat early in the day (yes, breakfast!), and finish as early as possible, too. Do the Five for Life Fast for an easy and effective method of time-restricted eating.

3. ***Eat the right food***. Most of all, this means *eat unprocessed food*. Lots of vegetables, plenty of protein and good fats. Use the Traffic Light Table and focus on eating mostly from the green zone. Notice what foods are in the red zone and danger zone, and begin to replace them, substituting from the amber and green zones.

4. ***Drink the right fluids***. Drink more water. Go easy on milk and caffeine. Avoid juices and sweetened drinks (including artificial sweeteners). Reduce alcohol. Try out green tea and vinegar.

5. ***Eat in the right way***. Eat slowly, with joy, gratitude and intention. Chew thoroughly before swallowing.

Part II looks at other factors that affect weight and weight gain:

- ***Micronutrients*** – the importance of getting enough of the right vitamins, minerals and polyphenols.

- ***Microbiome*** – the role of the happy gut, and how to increase your chances of having one.

- ***Metabolism*** – how it's affected by diet, exercise and muscle mass, and how to keep yours high.

- ***Stress and sleep*** – how poor sleep and too much stress contribute to weight gain, and how to help regulate the hormones cortisol and melatonin to your advantage.

- ***Shift work*** – how this perfect storm of stress and disrupted sleep leads to storage of abdominal fat, and what you can do about it.

- *Being female*! – the times in our lives when we're more prone to gaining excess weight, and suggestions for protective measures.

Part III is full of practical suggestions for using the Five for Life approach to tackle some of the everyday situations that seem to challenge our best intentions:

- *Navigating the day* – recognising trigger points for unhelpful eating, and some suggestions for strategies (including for snacking).

- *Getting meals on the table* – shopping and meal preparation are key to making better food choices easy.

- *Food advertising* – exposing the traps used by advertisers, debunking myths around the 'magic words' they use, and using nutritional labels to your advantage.

Where to start?

Where to start will be different for everyone. Maybe you're already a faithful breakfast eater, or drink a lot of water, so those habits won't need changing. But maybe you don't eat regularly, or you usually eat dinner at 8 pm, or in front of the TV (or both). Or maybe, *like more than 90% of Australians*, you don't manage five serves of veggies a day.

Hopefully, this book has helped identify your own most undermining habits. Acknowledge that these are part of your current lifestyle, and that it's right here that the small changes need to begin.

For the 'what to eat' bit, focus on what to eat *more of*, rather than what *not* to eat. Eat more quality protein and more vegetables, and eat more regularly. No-one's stopping you from eating red zone or danger zone food, but make it your first priority to get enough protein and 400 g of vegetables every day. You probably won't want to fit much more in on top of that.

Tackling *when* to eat is critical – and easily as important as 'what' to eat. The numerous breakfast studies and growing body of studies on time-restricted eating, show us eating in sync with our circadian rhythm is essential. If, like probably most of us, one of your main hurdles is going to be eating your last meal earlier, make it your focus to start doing the *Five for Life Fast* just once per week. On other days, work on eating as early as you can, and reducing the size of that last meal. Use the portion management and mindful eating techniques described in Chapters 3 and 6 to help get used to enjoying a much smaller serving in the evenings. If you work shifts, staying true to your circadian rhythm will be more difficult, but it's doable. Chapter 8 has some ideas to try.

Gently does it

This is not the 'battle of the bulge'. You're not going to war against your body, or even having an argument with it.

The route back to a healthy weight, for life, is to begin making changes in the way you think about food and eating. These will lead to changes in actions and, over time, small and consistent changes in daily eating habits will lead to healthier weight. Small changes allow your body to naturally re-set its sense of how much weight it needs to carry. Keep your focus on the positives that come with moving towards your ideal weight, in a sustainable way.

Let compassion be your guide, and seek out those who support you.

The Five for Life website has further resources.

Megan Dyson
Five for Life
www.5forlife.com.au

APPENDIX A

BEST CHOICES / WHAT TO EAT

BREAKFAST	
Have this	*... instead of this*
Eggs – any way you like them	Toast
Fish – e.g. salmon or sardines	Fruit juice (sweetened or unsweetened)
Bacon or sausages (go for butcher-made sausages with minimal fillers, and limit to not more than once per week)	Processed breakfast drinks (e.g. UP&GO™)
Always add plenty of vegetables to your protein – e.g. broccoli, kale, spinach, tomato or avocado	Any cereal-based processed 'breakfast food'
Plain rolled oats with unflavoured, unsweetened plain yoghurt, small quantity of berries and raw nuts or seeds (you'll need an additional source of protein to make a full breakfast)	Commercial breakfast cereal, including bran-based cereal (high in sugar despite its 'healthy' claims)
Add to your low-carb breakfast if you need more energy: a single piece of wholegrain bread or plain yoghurt	

LUNCH

Have this	... instead of this
Protein source with salad – plenty of non-starchy vegetables and pulses (chickpeas, black beans, lentils); dress with nuts or seeds, and home-made salad dressing Protein source with roast vegetables – carrots, pumpkin, swede, cauliflower and brussels sprouts; dress with home-made salad dressing. Small quantities of roast potato, sweet potato, sweet corn or beetroot are also fine If you're looking for crunch with your salad, use a sprinkle of mixed nuts and seeds: pepitas, sunflower kernels, and a few pine nuts makes a delicious mix. (Forget the crispy noodles, they're full of carbs and Omega-6 in the form of highly processed vegetable oil)	Sandwiches Wraps Pasta- or rice-based meals (including sushi) Anything shallow- or deep-fried Anything battered Anything in a pastry shell Noodles with your salad or veg

DINNER

Have this	... instead of this
Poached, baked, casseroled or stir-fried meat, poultry, seafood, tofu, tempeh or pulses with mixed non-starchy vegetables (roasted, steamed, fried or raw, and/or as a salad)	Pasta- or rice-based meal Pasta, rice, bread or potatoes as side dish Anything shallow- or deep-fried Anything battered Anything in a pastry shell

SNACKS
Find recipes for some of these on the Five for Life website

Have this	*... instead of this*
Canned fish	
Raw nuts or seeds	
Half an avocado	
Grain-free seed crackers	
Home-made dips – hummus, baba ganoush, tzatziki, carrot and cashew dip, cannellini bean dip, or avocado dip with vegetable sticks	Commercially-made dips – French onion dip, cashew dip, pesto dip etc
Lower-sugar fruit such as berries, citrus, kiwifruit or watermelon; add some plain yoghurt for a more substantial snack	Biscuits (savoury, for cheese or dips)
Dark chocolate (plain and very dark – at least 75% cocoa and sugar less than 18 g/100 g). Small piece only; 25–30 g max per day	Potato crisps Muesli bar Chips
Meat jerky (check sugar content; sometimes it's been sugar-cured before drying). Go for grass-fed beef or kangaroo, which contain more Omega-3 oils	Cake or biscuits Muffin (sweet or savoury)
Trail mix (yes you can add a small amount of 75% minimum cocoa dark chocolate, but *limit quantity*)	Protein balls (unless home-made, low sugar) Confectionery
Roasted chickpeas or fava/broad beans (watch out for sugar and vegetable oils; best make them yourself), seaweed wafers	Dried fruit Most types of chocolate
Hard boiled eggs – my favourite! Sanitary, safe, no mess, no cutlery required, shells are compostable	Any processed snacks
Peanut butter celery sticks	
Cottage cheese (plain or savoury – check label for additives) with raw veggie sticks	

Home-made protein bar/balls (*limit quantity*)	
Edamame beans (fresh or frozen)	
Plain yoghurt – mix with nuts, shredded dried coconut (unsweetened) and small quantity of berries	

BAKING	
Have this	*... instead of this*
Generally, make baking a special occasion thing only Reduce carb content of cake by: • reducing sugar to about half what the ingredients say (it doesn't affect the outcome, except for meringue) • using recipes with low-carb flour alternatives such as almond meal or coconut flour	Cake with wheat or gluten-free flour and sugar (any variety)

FOOD TYPES

Have this	*... instead of this*
Breakfast cereal Plain rolled oats or a low-sugar, oat-based muesli (note that even with plain yoghurt, oats for breakfast does not have enough protein to form a meal) *Limit oats and muesli to 35 g per serve*	Everything else
Cheese Cottage cheese, small quantities of soft cheese (e.g. brie, camembert), cheddar or hard cheese. Be aware of high fat (energy) content, as it's easy to overeat	Flavoured and processed cheese (e.g. cheese spread, flavoured cream cheese)
Crackers/biscuits Seed crackers made with psyllium husk	Biscuits made from refined-grain flour; any sweet biscuit
Fat Unprocessed plant fats and cold-pressed oils – avocado, olives, coconut, raw nuts and seeds Unprocessed animal fats – butter, cream, cheese *(limit quantities: saturated fats are likely to be more fattening than unrefined mono- and polyunsaturated fats)*	Refined and processed fats – margarine, hydrogenated vegetable oil, processed lard, trans fats, superheated or repeat-heated fats (e.g. from deep-fryers)
Fruit Low-sugar fruit, especially berries	Frequent serves of high-sugar fruit such as grapes, cherries, pears, figs, bananas, mango; dried fruit

Meat Unprocessed meat from any source	Processed meat from any source
Milk Full fat or reduced fat. Be aware of high energy content of full cream milk	Flavoured milk
Oil Cold-pressed natural vegetable oils – e.g. olive oil, coconut oil, macadamia oil, avocado oil	Processed vegetable oils such as sunflower, safflower, canola, and grapeseed oils
Preserved vegetables Fermented vegetables including sauerkraut, kimchi, other fermented vegetables Vegetables preserved in salt brine	Pickled vegetables – these have generally not been fermented, but are pickled in a mix of vinegar, herbs, spices *and sugar*
Vegetables All vegetables *(Limit quantities of starchy vegetables)*	Starchy vegetables processed with fats – e.g. frozen chips/nuggets, potato chips and crisps
Vinegar All vinegar, especially long-fermented, unfiltered vinegar like apple cider vinegar, aged rice vinegar or malt vinegar	Balsamic glaze – balsamic vinegar mixed with sugar or malt Shop-bought salad dressings
Yoghurt Plain unflavoured yoghurt – full fat or fat reduced *Check the label on non-dairy yoghurts. These are often highly processed, with ingredients that aren't included in plain, unflavoured yoghurt made from fermented dairy milk*	Flavoured yoghurt or yoghurt drinks

APPENDIX B

THE GLYCAEMIC INDEX

The glycaemic index (or GI) is a measurement of how quickly a particular food raises the level of glucose in our blood.[66] Pure fat or protein, or fat/protein combinations, have minimal effect on blood sugar, so they aren't included in the GI. The GI just measures food that's pure carbs, or includes carbs.

The GI is a scale of 0–100. The higher food is on the scale, the more quickly it raises blood sugar. For example, pure glucose has a GI of 100. White bread has a GI ranging from 70–90, while potatoes (depending on the variety) have a GI of over 95. Cooked kidney beans have a GI of 36. Very low-carb vegetables such as leafy greens have an estimated GI less than 5.

Carbohydrates with a high GI raise blood glucose very quickly. The higher the GI of a food, the higher our blood sugar and insulin will spike, causing us to store the excess energy as body fat. A spike in insulin brings blood sugar down quickly (as the energy is taken up by cells) and leads to a 'low' – often accompanied by cravings for more carbs. If we eat a lot of carbs at one sitting, especially if they're higher GI foods, the total glycaemic 'load' of the meal (that is, the overall effect on our blood sugar and demand on insulin) will also be high.

As high-GI carbs convert so quickly, we get a double whammy – even quicker conversion to glucose, and greater likelihood that energy will end up stored as fat.

So in general terms – *steer away from high-GI carbs.* We mostly eat too much of them.

---

[66] The GI was invented in Canada in 1981 to help diabetics control blood sugar. The GI Symbol was developed in Australia by the University of Sydney, and is now used across the world to certify whether food is low, medium or high GI.

Which carbohydrates have high GI?

It's difficult to estimate the GI of foods. We only know for sure the GI of foods that have been tested in a lab. Broadly, though, non-starchy vegetables and unprocessed pulses have low GI, whereas sugary and highly processed foods tend to have high to very high GI.

There are online tables showing the GI of different foods. I use the University of Sydney tables at https://glycemicindex.com/gi-search/.

The main high-GI carbs to look out for are:

- *Sugar* in all its forms
  - » For example, table sugar, honey, corn syrup, maple syrup
- *Processed starches*
  - » Bread! White bread has very high GI. Wholegrain bread generally has medium GI, while most sourdough is low
  - » Rice – there is little difference in GI of white vs. brown rice
  - » Processed breakfast cereals
- *Potatoes*.

Notice something? *All red zone carbs are high GI.* Potatoes, although in the amber zone, also have high GI. Many fruits (amber zone again) also have high GI.

Does low GI mean 'good'?

Not necessarily. Just because a food has a low GI doesn't mean it's 'good for you'. *Junk food will have a low GI if it also has a high fat content (e.g. chocolate, potato crisps).*[67] That's why I prefer to classify carbs as green, amber or red, and use the 'danger zone' to identify carbs that have been prepared in a way that's unheathy.

---

[67] Low GI is anything below 55. The GI of generic brand salted potato chips is 51. Milk chocolate is 42; dark chocolate is 23.

How to reduce GI

All green zone carbs have a very low GI.

Amber and red carbs have higher GI. You can reduce the GI a little, by changing the way you prepare them:

- Cook potatoes, pasta and rice, then refrigerate. This changes the chemical composition of the starches, making them more difficult to digest. The process means planning ahead, but it's a technique to consider if you *really* want that potato or pasta salad. While reheated rice and pasta seem to retain most of the altered starch structure, research indicates that in potatoes, starch returns to normal composition when reheated.

- Add vinegar or lemon juice to your meal, or have a glass of water mixed with two teaspoons of vinegar (apple cider or aged Chinese or Japanese rice vinegar are best) before or during your meal.

- Add a little salad dressing – oil and vinegar both slow down the speed at which blood sugar rises. Use home-made only, as manufactured salad dressings are usually loaded with sugar as well as other additives.

- Add fibre. The more fibre food has, the longer it takes for carbs in the meal to be converted into glucose. Unprocessed fibre (e.g. leafy greens like kale stalks!) does a better job at this.

- Reduce processing. The longer food is cooked (e.g. overdone pasta) or broken up (e.g. mashing potatoes or using quick oats instead of rolled oats), the higher its GI will be.

Although reducing GI means a slower rise in blood sugar, there will still be a rise. Any sugar we don't need straight away is converted and stored, mostly as fat.

APPENDIX C

SIMPLE GUIDE TO MEAL-BUILDING

This *Five for Life* guide to meal-building or meal planning is based on having three to five small meals per day. The principles are the same for every meal:

1. Protein first

2. Then non-starchy vegetables

3. Then fat (there might already be enough in the protein source)

4. Amber zone carbs if you need them.

Let's use my friend Maireana as an example. Maireana wants to reduce her body fat without losing muscle mass or feeling low in energy.

1. ***Calculate daily protein needs.*** This is around 1.2–1.5 grams per kilo of your body weight, per day.

> *Maireana weighs 70 kg, so she's aiming to have 85–100 g protein per day.*

2. ***Share it out.*** Divide total daily protein requirements into individual meals and snacks. If you have milk in your tea or coffee, count this as a snack too (a 250 ml cows-milk coffee, made latte style, is about 7–8 g of protein. For dairy substitutes, check the protein content on the nutrition label). For smaller meals, aim for 20 g of protein. Larger meals can be 20–30 g.

> *Maireana likes to have three meals, and two flat white coffees, per day. She snacks on almonds and plain yoghurt, as well as vegetables and fruit.*
>
> *Milk in the coffee counts for about 15 g protein, with 10 g protein in the nuts and yoghurt. This means Maireana needs 60–75 g protein from her meals. That's three meals of approximately 20–25 g protein each.*

4. *Pick your protein.* For each meal – decide on your **main source of protein**. Have a look online for examples of what 20–30 g of protein looks like. It doesn't need to be precise; close enough is good enough. The Five for Life website has a downloadable table of common protein sources.

> *Maireana prefers eggs, fish and chicken for her main protein sources, but she also loves the creamy texture of black beans.*
>
> *A couple of large eggs have about 15 g protein. Fish has about 22 g protein per 100 g. Chicken breast has 35 g protein per 100 g. Two eggs, or a piece of chicken approximately the size of her palm, or a small can of fish, will give Maireana nearly all she needs for a meal.*
>
> *There's also protein in pulses (about 5 g protein per half cup) and cheese (6 g protein in a chunk about the size of your thumb).*

5. *Vibrant veggies.* Have one to two loosely clenched fistfuls of cooked or raw non-starchy vegetables with each main meal.

> *Maireana loves crisp salad greens and cucumber, sweet capsicum, tomatoes and crunchy green beans. And broccoli and kale quickly fried in a hot pan with a little olive oil, finished with a tablespoon of boiling water to steam them through.*

6. *Fat to fit.* Use cold-pressed olive, avocado or nut oil, fish, or olives, raw nuts or seeds. You don't need much – about a tablespoon of nuts or seeds, or a quarter of an avocado, or a few olives, or a couple of teaspoons of oil in a dressing. If your protein source contains a lot

of fat (e.g. eggs, lamb, smoked salmon or canned tuna in olive oil), or you've used fat in cooking, or in salad or vegetable dressings, you might not need much extra.

> *Maireana drizzles pretty much everything with her home-made olive oil and vinegar dressing. She also keeps a jar of mixed seeds in the fridge to sprinkle on salads for extra taste and texture. She uses olive oil to stir-fry.*

7. ***(Maybe) add some green or amber zone carbs.*** For meals before 3 pm, add a small cupped handful. If your protein source is pulses, or this is your last meal of the day, leave out these extra carbs.

Maireana's Monday

This sample meal plan provides about 1,500 calories, with plenty of vegetables and approximately 90 g protein, 100 g carbs and 70 g fat, all from high-quality sources.

The numbers in brackets are protein estimates for each item.

> *Breakfast at 7.30 am*
> *Flat white coffee (7 g), two large poached eggs (15 g), 1 cup of steamed kale and broccoli (2 g) and a piece of sourdough toast (3 g)*
>
> *Morning snack at 10 am*
> *Handful of almonds (5 g), an orange and another coffee (7 g)*
>
> *Lunch at 12 noon*
> *Small can of tuna (15 g) with half a cup of black beans (5 g), a small cupped handful of quinoa and wild rice (2 g) and 2 cups of salad greens, avocado, tomatoes and cucumber with pepper, olive oil, vinegar and Dijon mustard*
>
> *Afternoon snack at 2 pm*
> *Quarter cup of frozen blueberries with a cup of plain yoghurt (6 g)*
>
> *Dinner at 6.30 pm*
> *Chicken breast (a piece the size of her palm) (22 g) with stir-fried vegetables (5 g)*

On days Maireana does her *Five for Life Fast*, she brings lunch forward to 11.30, and eats her dinner meal at 3.30–4 pm.

Sometimes she combines her morning snack and lunch at 11 am and has her main meal in the early afternoon, then fruit and yoghurt at 6 pm as a light last morsel. This way of eating isn't quite as effective as the longer overnight fast, but it still cuts down the amount to be digested before bed and is an easy way to reduce evening eating while still having all necessary nutrients.

ACKNOWLEDGEMENTS

My heartfelt gratitude to the many people who contributed their thoughts and encouragement throughout this project, as the book would not exist but for you.

In particular, Peter Hoey, Annette Davison, Hayley Davis, Rosemary Argue, Gaby Jaksa, Lucy and Colin, who generously read drafts and provided numerous insightful comments and suggestions.

Special thanks to Annette for your friendship, support, positive energy and imagination, and for being such a generous sounding board throughout. I deeply appreciate the numerous hours you carved out of your own impossible schedule for me.

Peter, thank you for pushing and never doubting me; you've been a wonderful mentor in both my careers.

Lucy, thank you for your joyful photography, yoga, love and unwavering faith despite my insecurities and hand-wringing. My sister Fiona, I'm so grateful for your keen design eye and wise advice on all manner of things.

Maria Panagiotidis, thank you for seeding the idea for this book!

For the nuts and bolts – thank you to Rob Clode for the striking Five for Life icons. Amy Lovat for empathetic editing and Sally Asnicar for additional editing and eagle-eyed proof-reading. And Tess McCabe for your skill, patience and professionalism with the book design, as well as advice about many other aspects of book production and publishing.

And to Colin, Stuart and James – for your love, and for supporting me in spending all my spare time on this project and putting up with me going on a lot about vegetables.

GLOSSARY

Ancient grains

Ancient grains are grains used by our ancestors before modern grains such as wheat became more common in the Western diet. They're still a staple of diets in many other parts of the world. They include quinoa, millet, freekeh, spelt and wild rice.

Body fat/fat cells

Body fat, or adipose tissue, is our body's own stores of fat. We need to be carrying some body fat, but too much puts us at risk of serious health problems.

Calories

A calorie is a unit of energy. We use calories to measure the amount of fuel for our body that is provided by an item of food. For example, one medium egg gives us around 75 calories. Another unit to measure food energy is the kilojoule (kJ) – there are about 4.2 kJ to a calorie. I use calories in this book.

Carbohydrates/carbs

Carbohydrates (or carbs) are fibres, sugars and starches. We normally don't include fibre when we discuss carbs, as fibre passes through the body mostly undigested.

Sugars and starches are an important source of energy, because our body metabolises them quickly into glucose. If we don't use that glucose for energy straight away, our body converts it and converts it to store as body fat.

In this book, carb-containing foods are classified by a 'traffic light' system:

- Green zone: Unlimited – get most of your carbs from these foods
- Amber zone: Treat with caution – it's fine to get some of your carbs from these foods
- Red zone: Avoid – it's not healthy to have your carbs from these foods.

In this book, food is counted as high in carbs if at least 50% of its energy value comes from starch or sugar. The Traffic Light Table for Carbs on page 134 lists high-carb foods.

Circadian rhythm

Circadian rhythm is our internal body clock. It controls a variety of bodily systems, including our metabolism, and a disrupted circadian rhythm is strongly associated with overweight and obesity. Eating at night-time disrupts our circadian rhythm, causing changes to metabolism that lead to weight gain.

Eating in sync with our circadian rhythm helps us shed fat, and keep it off.

Danger zone food

This is my term for food that is a potent, hyper-tasty mix of carbs, fat and added sugar and/or salt. Danger zone foods are a red flag. Eating them undermines our efforts to reach and stay at a happy weight.

Dietary fat

Dietary fat is the fat that we eat – for example, in oils, nuts and seeds, and in animal products like eggs, milk and meat. It's an essential part of our diet but there are different types of fats, some better for us than others. This book uses a traffic light system to help choose the best fats.

Discretionary food

This is a 'health-wash' term used by the junk food and confectionery industry, and in government dietary guidelines, for food our bodies don't need. In other words, filler food.

FODMAPs

FODMAPs is an acronym for types of carbs that ferment in our gut: Fermentable Oligosaccharides, Disaccharides, Monosaccharides And Polyols. FODMAPs can upset the digestive systems of people sensitive to them.

Fruit

In this book, fruit means the sweet-tasting parts of plants that we normally call fruit, such as apples, pears, bananas etc. Technically, fruit is the product of the flower of a plant that contains seeds. Many vegetables are actually fruit, including avocados, tomatoes, pumpkins, eggplants, zucchini and legumes, but we normally refer to them as vegetables.

Glycaemic Index (GI)

The glycaemic index (or GI) is a measurement of how easy it is for our body to turn different carbs into glucose. The GI is a scale of 0–100. The higher food is on the scale, the more quickly it raises our blood sugar (not a good thing). Generally, it's best to choose food that is low GI. Appendix B has more on the GI.

Glycaemic Load (GL)

Glycaemic load (GL) is a measure of how much our blood sugar rises because of the combination of total carbs and GI of those carbs, eaten in a single sitting.

Gut microbiome

The gut microbiome is the community of micro-organisms that live in our gut – in their trillions. For our best health, we need them in a high level of diversity and abundance. An unhappy microbiome has a significant impact on our health, including our weight.

High-quality carbs

High-quality carbs are unprocessed or have had only minimal processing, and are high in fibre. Unprocessed vegetables, fruits and whole grains (green zone and amber zone foods) are high-quality carbs.

Low-GI carbs

Low-GI carbs have a lower impact on our blood sugar, which is a good thing. While most low-GI carbs are green or amber zone foods, some are in the red or danger zone, because low GI does not necessarily mean 'good for you'. Appendix B has more about the GI.

Low-quality/low-value carbs

Low-quality carbs are the opposite of high-quality carbs. Low-quality carbs have usually been refined to remove all but the starch or sugar component of the original plant, and are found in most highly processed foods. They include white rice and refined flour (including most gluten-free flours) and are categorised as red zone foods. The Traffic Light Table for Carbs on page 134 lists the main sources of low-quality carbs.

Macronutrients

Macronutrients are the nutrients that provide us with energy (calories). The four macronutrients are carbohydrates, protein, fat and alcohol. Chapter 4 explains what protein, fat and carbs are. Alcohol, not a macronutrient our bodies need, is discussed in Chapter 5.

Metabolic rate

Metabolic rate is the rate at which our bodies burn energy, while resting and while exercising. Metabolic rate is individual to each person, but can be estimated through a formula that takes into account sex, weight, height and age.

People with a high resting metabolic rate ('fast metabolism') burn energy more quickly than people with a low resting metabolic rate ('slow metabolism'). What and how we eat can alter our metabolism; see more in Chapter 7.

Metabolic health

Good metabolic health means having appropriate fasting blood sugar, low blood lipids (triglycerides and low-density cholesterol), good blood pressure and a safe waist circumference. Poor metabolic health directly increases the risk of heart disease, diabetes and stroke.

Metabolic syndrome

Metabolic syndrome is a cluster of symptoms, including high blood pressure, high LDL cholesterol or low HDL cholesterol, high blood sugar and abdominal obesity.

Micronutrients

Micronutrients are the vitamins, minerals and trace elements that are essential for our bodies to function properly, even though we need them only in tiny amounts.

Nutrient dense

Nutrient-dense (nutrient-rich) food is high in micronutrients, protein and/or 'good' fat. For example, unprocessed meat, seafood, vegetables and fruit are nutrient dense. Red zone and danger zone food is not.

Obesogenic

Obesogenic means 'tending to cause obesity'. An obesogenic environment promotes weight gain, in the sense that it surrounds us with influences and pressures that discourage physical activity and healthy diets, such as excessive access to unhealthy foods and food advertising, sedentary lifestyles and shift work.

Prebiotics

Prebiotics are non-digestible substances – essentially, fibre – that 'feed' good gut microbes. Fibre in vegetables, fruit, oats, pulses and psyllium are prebiotics.

Probiotics

Probiotics are the 'good' microbes in our gut, but the word is more commonly used to refer to foods that contain probiotics. The more probiotics in our gut, of a greater variety, the healthier we will be.

Fermented foods contain high levels of probiotics – yoghurt, sauerkraut and kimchi, tempeh and miso.

Processed food

Processed food is food that's not in its natural state. Processing can range from minimal (e.g. cutting and cooking or fermenting), right through to deconstruction and artificial ingredients. When we talk about processed food being unhealthy, we're talking about food that has been subjected to more than just cooking or fermenting.

Highly processed foods are a risk to our health. A simple test is to check the label. If the item couldn't be made in a kitchen, with ordinary ingredients from a food market, it's highly processed.

Psyllium husk

Psyllium husk is the outer layer of a type of grass seed. Usually just called psyllium, it is a common and effective dietary fibre supplement.

Pulses (dried beans)

Pulses are the edible seeds inside the pods of legumes. They're normally dried before eating, and include kidney beans, butter beans, black beans, pinto beans, split peas, chickpeas, lentils and edamame (fresh soy) beans. Pulses are high in fibre and an important source of protein.

Pulses are sometimes referred to as legumes, even though they're not. Legumes are the whole plants whose seeds and seed pods we eat, such as snow peas and green beans.

Starchy vegetables

All vegetables contain some carbs – fibre, sugar and/or starch. Some are particularly high in starch, but most are not.

Starchy vegetables are potatoes, sweet potatoes, sweet corn, parsnips, garden peas and pumpkins. Out of these, potatoes have by far the most starch, followed by sweet potato and sweet corn. As starch is a type of carb, starchy vegetables are also much higher in carbs overall than non-starchy vegetables.

Non-starchy vegetables are all the other ones.

Thermic effect of food (diet-induced thermogenesis)

When we eat anything, our body uses energy to digest it. This is called the 'thermic effect' of food, and it's part of what makes up our metabolism. Some foods (e.g. foods high in protein) have a higher thermic effect than others.

Visceral fat

Visceral fat is the deep belly fat that collects around our internal organs, with significant negative health impacts. It is also known as 'toxic fat' because it produces hormones and other chemicals that travel through the bloodstream, increasing our risk of serious illness, including heart disease, type 2 diabetes and some cancers. Visceral fat is a significant breast cancer risk, and this risk grows significantly higher after menopause.

Weight

Our weight is made up of fat, muscle, bone, water, blood and organs. In this book, 'weight' in the context of reducing weight means the part of our weight that is body fat.

Weight 'set point'

Our weight set point is our body's innate sense of the right weight for us. It's easy to move the set point up, but difficult and slow to move it down.

REFERENCES

Five for Life is based on numerous studies and reviews reported in peer-reviewed scientific journals. This chapter lists some of the key sources. Sources marked with an asterisk are studies used as specific examples in the chapter text.

CHAPTER ONE. CHANGING HABITS

Cleo, G. et al. (2019). Habit-based interventions for weight loss maintenance in adults with overweight and obesity: a randomized controlled trial. *International journal of obesity (2005), 43*(2), 374–383. https://doi.org/10.1038/s41366-018-0067-4

Gardner, B. et al. (2012). Making health habitual: the psychology of 'habit-formation' and general practice. *The British journal of general practice : the journal of the Royal College of General Practitioners, 62*(605), 664–666. https://doi.org/10.3399/bjgp12X659466

Gardner, B. et al. (2014). Putting habit into practice, and practice into habit: a process evaluation and exploration of the acceptability of a habit-based dietary behaviour change intervention. *International journal of behavioral nutrition and physical activity 11* (135). https://doi.org/10.1186/s12966-014-0135-7

CHAPTER TWO. TREASURE YOUR BODY

Power of words

Patrick, V., & Hagtvedt, H. (2012). "I don't" versus "I can't": When empowered refusal motivates goal-directed behavior. *Journal of consumer research, 39*(2), 371–381. https://doi.org/10.1086/663212

Obesogenicity

*Australian Institute of Health and Welfare. (2020) *Overweight and obesity: an interactive insight.* Australian Government available online https://www.aihw.gov.au/reports/overweight-obesity/overweight-and-obesity-an-interactive-insight/contents/what-is-overweight-and-obesity

Gupta, R. et al. (2020). Endocrine disruption and obesity: A current review on environmental obesogens. *Current research in green and sustainable chemistry. 3*(2020), 100009, ISSN 2666-0865, https://doi.org/10.1016/j.crgsc.2020.06.002

Leaf, A. & Antonio, J. (2017). The effects of overfeeding on body composition: the role of macronutrient composition - a narrative review. *International journal of exercise science, 10*(8), 1275–1296. https://www.ncbi.nlm.nih.gov/pmc/articles/PMC5786199/

Jenkinson, A. (2020) *Why we eat (too much): The new science of appetite.* Penguin (2020)

Visceral fat

Iyengar, N. et al. (2019). Association of body fat and risk of breast cancer in postmenopausal women with normal body mass index: a secondary analysis of a randomized clinical trial and observational study. *JAMA oncology, 5*(2), 155–163. https://doi.org/10.1001/jamaoncol.2018.5327

Shuster, A. et al. (2012). The clinical importance of visceral adiposity: a critical review of methods for visceral adipose tissue analysis. *The British journal of radiology, 85*(1009), 1–10. https://doi.org/10.1259/bjr/38447238

Hou, J. et al. (2020). Obesity and bone health: a complex link. *Frontiers in cell and developmental biology, 8,* 600181. https://doi.org/10.3389/fcell.2020.600181

Turcotte, A. et al. (2021) Association between obesity and risk of fracture, bone mineral density and bone quality in adults: A systematic review and meta-analysis. *PLoS ONE 16*(6): e0252487 https://doi.org/10.1371/journal.pone.0252487

Després, J., & Lemieux, I. (2006). Abdominal obesity and metabolic syndrome. *Nature, 444*(7121), 881–887. https://doi.org/10.1038/nature05488

Diabetes UK (2019). Visceral fat (active fat): https://www.diabetes.co.uk/body/visceral-fat.html

Self-weighing as a tool in weight management

VanWormer, J. et al. (2012). Self-weighing frequency is associated with weight gain prevention over 2 years among working adults. *International journal of behavioral medicine, 19*(3), 351–358. https://doi.org/10.1007/s12529-011-9178-1

Vuorinen, A. et al. (2021). Frequency of self-weighing and weight change: cohort study with 10,000 smart scale users. *Journal of medical Internet research, 23*(6), e25529. https://doi.org/10.2196/25529

Eating vs. exercise

Bellicha, A. (2021). Effect of exercise training on weight loss, body composition changes, and weight maintenance in adults with overweight or obesity: An overview of 12 systematic reviews and 149 studies. *Obesity reviews : an official journal of the International Association for the Study of Obesity, 22 Suppl 4,* e13256. https://doi.org/10.1111/obr.13256

MacKenzie-Shalders, K. et al. (2020). The effect of exercise interventions on resting metabolic rate: A systematic review and meta-analysis. *Journal of sports sciences, 38*(14), 1635–1649. https://doi.org/10.1080/02640414.2020.1754716

Schwingshackl, L. et al. (2014). Impact of long-term lifestyle programmes on weight loss and cardiovascular risk factors in overweight/obese participants: a systematic review and network meta-analysis. *Systematic reviews, 3,* 130. https://doi.org/10.1186/2046-4053-3-130

Swift, D. et al. (2014). The role of exercise and physical activity in weight loss and maintenance. *Progress in cardiovascular diseases, 56*(4), 441–447. https://doi.org/10.1016/j.pcad.2013.09.012

Westerterp, K. (2019). Physical activity and body-weight regulation. *The American journal of clinical nutrition 110*(4), 791-792. https://doi.org/10.1093/ajcn/nqz132

Westerterp, K. (2019). Control of energy expenditure in humans. [Updated 2019 Jul 25]. In: K. Feingold (Eds) et al. *Endotext* [Internet]. MDText.com, Inc. https://www.ncbi.nlm.nih.gov/books/NBK278963/

Posture

Mari, A. et al. (2019). Bloating and abdominal distension - clinical approach and management. *Advances in therapy, 36* (5):1075-1084. https://doi.org/10.1007/s12325-019-00924-7

Miles-Chan, J., & Dulloo, A. (2017). Posture allocation revisited: breaking the sedentary threshold of energy expenditure for obesity management. *Frontiers in physiology, 8,* 420. https://doi.org/10.3389/fphys.2017.00420

CHAPTER THREE. WHEN TO EAT

The stretched stomach

Geliebter, A. et al. (1996). Reduced stomach capacity in obese subjects after dieting. *The American journal of clinical nutrition, 63*(2), 170–173. https://doi.org/10.1093/ajcn/63.2.170

Portion sizes

Buettner, D. (2008). The Blue Zones: lessons for living longer from the people who've lived the longest. *Am J Lifestyle Med. 2016* Sep-Oct; 10(5): 318–321. https://journals.sagepub.com/doi/abs/10.1177/1559827616637066

Freedman, M. R., & Brochado, C. (2010). Reducing portion size reduces food intake and plate waste. *Obesity (Silver Spring, Md.), 18*(9), 1864–1866. https://doi.org/10.1038/oby.2009.480

Robinson, E., & Kersbergen, I. (2018). Portion size and later food intake: evidence on the "normalizing" effect of reducing food portion sizes. *The American journal of clinical nutrition, 107*(4), 640–646, https://doi.org/10.1093/ajcn/nqy013

Sheen, F. et al. (2018). Plate-clearing tendencies and portion size are independently associated with main meal food intake in women: a laboratory study. *Appetite, 127,* 223–229. https://doi.org/10.1016/j.appet.2018.04.020

Zlatevska, N. et al. (2014). Sizing up the effect of portion size on consumption: a meta-analytic review. *Journal of marketing, 78*(3), 140–154. https://doi.org/10.1509/jm.12.0303

Zuraikat, F. et al. (2018). Doggy bags and downsizing: packaging uneaten food to go after a meal attenuates the portion size effect in women. *Appetite, 129*, 162–170. https://doi.org/10.1016/j.appet.2018.07.009

Using portion control tools

Vargas-Alvarez, M. et al. (2021). Impact of portion control tools on portion size awareness, choice and intake: systematic review and meta-analysis. *Nutrients, 13*(6), 1978. https://doi.org/10.3390/nu13061978

Eat regularly

Paoli, A. et al. (2019). The influence of meal frequency and timing on health in humans: the role of fasting. *Nutrients, 11*(4), 719. https://www.mdpi.com/2072-6643/11/4/719

Pot, G. (2018). Sleep and dietary habits in the urban environment: the role of chrono-nutrition. *The Proceedings of the Nutrition Society, 77*(3), 189–198. https://doi.org/10.1017/S0029665117003974

Pot, G. et al (2016). Irregularity of energy intake at meals: prospective associations with the metabolic syndrome in adults of the 1946 British birth cohort. *The British journal of nutrition, 115*(2), 315–323. https://doi.org/10.1017/S0007114515004407

St-Onge, M. et al (2017). Meal timing and frequency: implications for cardiovascular disease prevention: a scientific statement from the American Heart Association. *Circulation, 135*(9), e96–e121. https://doi.org/10.1161/CIR.0000000000000476

Timlin, M., & Pereira, M. (2007). Breakfast frequency and quality in the etiology of adult obesity and chronic diseases. *Nutrition reviews, 65*(6 Pt 1), 268–281. https://doi.org/10.1301/nr.2007.jun.268-281

Eat in time with your circadian rhythm: Eat early (breakfast, and most calories in the earlier part of the day)

Randomised controlled trials and clinical studies

Bandín, C. et al. (2015). Meal timing affects glucose tolerance, substrate oxidation and circadian-related variables: A randomized, crossover trial. *International journal of obesity (2015), 39*(5), 828–833. https://doi.org/10.1038/ijo.2014.182

Betts, J. et al (2014). The causal role of breakfast in energy balance and health: a randomized controlled trial in lean adults. *The American journal of clinical nutrition, 100*(2), 539–547. https://doi.org/10.3945/ajcn.114.083402

Bo, S. et al. (2015). Is the timing of caloric intake associated with variation in diet-induced thermogenesis and in the metabolic pattern? A randomized cross-over study. *International journal of obesity (2005), 39*(12), 1689–1695. https://doi.org/10.1038/ijo.2015.138

Chowdhury, E. et al. (2016) The causal role of breakfast in energy balance and health: a randomized controlled trial in obese adults. *The American journal of clinical nutrition, 103*(3), 747–756. https://doi.org/10.3945/ajcn.115.122044

Garaulet, M. et al. (2013). Timing of food intake predicts weight loss effectiveness. *International journal of obesity (2005)*, 37(4), 604–611. https://www.nature.com/articles/ijo2012229

Hutchison, A. et al. (2019). Time-restricted feeding improves glucose tolerance in men at risk for type 2 diabetes: a randomized crossover trial. *Obesity (Silver Spring, Md.)*, 27(5), 724–732. https://doi.org/10.1002/oby.22449

Jakubowicz, D. et al. (2013). High caloric intake at breakfast vs. dinner differentially influences weight loss of overweight and obese women. *Obesity (Silver Spring, Md.)*, 21(12), 2504–2512. https://doi.org/10.1002/oby.20460

Jakubowicz, D. et al. (2015). Fasting until noon triggers increased postprandial hyperglycemia and impaired insulin response after lunch and dinner in individuals with type 2 diabetes: a randomized clinical trial. *Diabetes care, 38*(10), 1820–1826. https://doi.org/10.2337/dc15-0761

*Kelly, K. et al. (2020). Eating breakfast and avoiding late-evening snacking sustains lipid oxidation. *PLoS biology, 18*(2), e3000622. https://doi.org/10.1371/journal.pbio.3000622

Kessler, K. et al. (2017). The effect of diurnal distribution of carbohydrates and fat on glycaemic control in humans: a randomized controlled trial. *Scientific reports, 7,* 44170. https://doi.org/10.1038/srep44170

Lowe, D. et al. (2020). Effects of time-restricted eating on weight loss and other metabolic parameters in women and men with overweight and obesity: The TREAT randomized clinical trial. *JAMA internal medicine, 180*(11), 1491–1499. https://doi.org/10.1001/jamainternmed.2020.4153

McHill, A. et al. (2017). Later circadian timing of food intake is associated with increased body fat. *The American journal of clinical nutrition, 106*(5), 1213–1219. https://pubmed.ncbi.nlm.nih.gov/28877894/

Przulj, D. et al. (2021). Time restricted eating as a weight loss intervention in adults with obesity. *PLoS ONE 16*(1): e0246186. https://doi.org/10.1371/journal.pone.0246186

Richter, J. et al (2020). Twice as high diet-induced thermogenesis after breakfast vs dinner on high-calorie as well as low-calorie meals. *The Journal of clinical endocrinology and metabolism, 105*(3), dgz311. https://doi.org/10.1210/clinem/dgz311

Scheer, F. et al. (2013). The internal circadian clock increases hunger and appetite in the evening independent of food intake and other behaviors. *Obesity (Silver Spring, Md.)*, 21(3), 421–423. https://doi.org/10.1002/oby.20351

Sutton, E. et al (2018). Early time-restricted feeding improves insulin sensitivity, blood pressure, and oxidative stress even without weight loss in men with prediabetes. *Cell metabolism, 27*(6), 1212–1221.e3. https://doi.org/10.1016/j.cmet.2018.04.010

Thomas, E. et al. (2020). Later meal and sleep timing predicts higher percent body fat. *Nutrients, 13*(1), 73. https://doi.org/10.3390/nu13010073

Xiao, Q. et al. (2021). The association between overnight fasting and body mass index in older adults: the interaction between duration and timing. *International journal of obesity (2005), 45*(3), 555–564. https://doi.org/10.1038/s41366-020-00715-z

Zitting, K. et al. (2018). Human resting energy expenditure varies with circadian phase. *Current biology: CB, 28*(22), 3685–3690.e3. https://doi.org/10.1016/j.cub.2018.10.005

Cohort studies

Almoosawi, S. et al. (2013). Time-of-day and nutrient composition of eating occasions: prospective association with the metabolic syndrome in the 1946 British birth cohort. *International journal of obesity (2005), 37*(5), 725–731. https://doi.org/10.1038/ijo.2012.103

Bo, S. et al. (2014). Consuming more of daily caloric intake at dinner predisposes to obesity. A 6-year population-based prospective cohort study. *PLoS ONE, 9*(9), e108467. https://doi.org/10.1371/journal.pone.0108467

Kahleova, H. et al. (2017). Meal frequency and timing are associated with changes in body mass index in Adventist Health Study 2. *The Journal of nutrition, 147*(9), 1722–1728. https://doi.org/10.3945/jn.116.244749

Pot, G. et al (2016). Irregularity of energy intake at meals: prospective associations with the metabolic syndrome in adults of the 1946 British birth cohort. *The British journal of nutrition, 115*(2), 315–323. https://doi.org/10.1017/S0007114515004407

Systematic reviews and meta-analyses

Adafer, R. et al. (2020). Food timing, circadian rhythm and chrononutrition: a systematic review of time-restricted eating's effects on human health. *Nutrients 2020, 12,* 3770. https://doi.org/10.3390/nu12123770

Ballon, A. et al. (2019). Breakfast skipping is associated with increased risk of type 2 diabetes among adults: a systematic review and meta-analysis of prospective cohort studies. *The Journal of nutrition, 149*(1), 106–113. https://doi.org/10.1093/jn/nxy194

Bonnet, J. et al. (2020). Breakfast skipping, body composition, and cardiometabolic risk: a systematic review and meta-analysis of randomized trials. *Obesity (Silver Spring, Md.), 28*(6), 1098–1109. https://doi.org/10.1002/oby.22791

Charlot, A. et al. (2021). Beneficial effects of early time-restricted feeding on metabolic diseases: importance of aligning food habits with the circadian clock. *Nutrients, 13*(5), 1405. https://doi.org/10.3390/nu13051405

Gwin, J. & Leidy, H. (2018). A review of the evidence surrounding the effects of breakfast consumption on mechanisms of weight management. *Advances in nutrition (Bethesda, Md.), 9*(6), 717–725. https://doi.org/10.1093/advances/nmy047

Jakubowicz, D. et al. (2021). Role of high energy breakfast "big breakfast diet" in clock gene regulation of postprandial hyperglycemia and weight loss in type 2 diabetes. *Nutrients, 13*(5), 1558. https://doi.org/10.3390/nu13051558

Kessler, K., & Pivovarova-Ramich, O. (2019). Meal timing, aging, and metabolic health. *International journal of molecular sciences, 20*(8), 1911. https://doi.org/10.3390/ijms20081911

Ma, X. et al. (2020). Skipping breakfast is associated with overweight and obesity: A systematic review and meta-analysis. *Obesity research & clinical practice, 14*(1), 1–8. https://doi.org/10.1016/j.orcp.2019.12.002

McHill, A. & Wright, K. (2017). Role of sleep and circadian disruption on energy expenditure and in metabolic predisposition to human obesity and metabolic disease. *Obesity reviews : an official journal of the International Association for the Study of Obesity, 18 Suppl 1*, 15–24. https://doi.org/10.1111/obr.12503

Noh, J. (2018). The effect of circadian and sleep disruptions on obesity risk. *Journal of obesity & metabolic syndrome, 27*(2), 78–83. https://doi.org/10.7570/jomes.2018.27.2.78

Paoli, A. et al. (2019). The influence of meal frequency and timing on health in humans: the role of fasting. *Nutrients, 11*(4), 719. https://doi.org/10.3390/nu11040719

Pickel, L., & Sung, H. (2020). Feeding rhythms and the circadian regulation of metabolism. *Frontiers in nutrition, 7*, 39. https://doi.org/10.3389/fnut.2020.00039

Pot, G. (2018). Sleep and dietary habits in the urban environment: the role of chrono-nutrition. *The Proceedings of the Nutrition Society, 77*(3), 189–198. https://doi.org/10.1017/S0029665117003974

Shaw, E. et al. (2019). The impact of time of day on energy expenditure: implications for long-term energy balance. *Nutrients, 11*(10):2383. https://doi.org/10.3390/nu11102383

St-Onge, M. et al. (2017). Meal timing and frequency: implications for cardiovascular disease prevention: a scientific statement from the American Heart Association. *Circulation, 135*(9), e96–e121. https://doi.org/10.1161/CIR.0000000000000476

Vaughan, K., & Mattison, J. (2018). Watch the clock, not the scale. *Cell metabolism, 27*(6), 1159–1160. https://doi.org/10.1016/j.cmet.2018.05.016

Wicherski, J. et al. (2021). Association between breakfast skipping and body weight: a systematic review and meta-analysis of observational longitudinal studies. *Nutrients, 13*(1), 272. https://doi.org/10.3390/nu13010272

Benefits of a high-protein, high-fibre breakfast

Clark, C. et al. (2006). Effects of breakfast meal composition on second meal metabolic responses in adults with type 2 diabetes mellitus. *European journal of clinical nutrition, 60*(9), 1122–1129. https://doi.org/10.1038/sj.ejcn.1602427

Brum, J. et al. (2016). Satiety effects of psyllium in healthy volunteers. *Appetite, 105*, 27–36. https://doi.org/10.1016/j.appet.2016.04.041

Jakubowicz, D. et al. (2013). High caloric intake at breakfast vs. dinner differentially influences weight loss of overweight and obese women. *Obesity (Silver Spring, Md.), 21*(12), 2504–2512. https://doi.org/10.1002/oby.20460

Hoertel, H. et al. (2014). A randomized crossover, pilot study examining the effects of a normal protein vs. high protein breakfast on food cravings and reward signals in overweight/obese "breakfast skipping", late-adolescent girls. *Nutrition journal 13*, 80. https://doi.org/10.1186/1475-2891-13-80

Exercising in the morning when fasted

*Barutcu, A. et al. (2021). Planned morning aerobic exercise in a fasted state increases energy intake in the preceding 24 h. *European journal of nutrition, 60*(6), 3387-3396. https://www.ncbi.nlm.nih.gov/pmc/articles/PMC8354893/

Benefits of ketogenesis

Gershuni, V. et al. (2018). Nutritional ketosis for weight management and reversal of metabolic syndrome. *Current nutrition reports, 7*(3), 97–106. https://doi.org/10.1007/s13668-018-0235-0

Effects of Very Low Calorie Diets (VLCD)

Fothergill, E. et al. (2016). Persistent metabolic adaptation 6 years after "The Biggest Loser" competition. *Obesity (Silver Spring, Md.), 24*(8), 1612–1619. https://doi.org/10.1002/oby.21538

Flanagan, E. et al. (2020). Calorie restriction and aging in humans. *Annual Review of Nutrition 2020 40*:1, 105-133 https://www.annualreviews.org/doi/full/10.1146/annurev-nutr-122319-034601

CHAPTER FOUR. WHAT TO EAT

Ultra-processed food is associated with weight gain and disease

Elizabeth, L. et al. (2020). Ultra-processed foods and health outcomes: a narrative review. *Nutrients, 12*(7), 1955. https://doi.org/10.3390/nu12071955

*Hall, K. et al. (2019). Ultra-processed diets cause excess calorie intake and weight gain: an inpatient randomized controlled trial of ad libitum food intake. *Cell metabolism, 32*,(4). https://doi.org/10.1016/j.cmet.2019.05.008

Protein

Acheson, K. et al. (2011). Protein choices targeting thermogenesis and metabolism. *The American journal of clinical nutrition, 93*(3), 525–534. https://doi.org/10.3945/ajcn.110.005850

Anton, S. et al. (2018). Nutrition and exercise in sarcopenia. *Current protein & peptide science, 19*(7), 649–667. https://doi.org/10.2174/1389203717666161227144349

Arentson-Lantz, E. et al. (2015). Protein: A nutrient in focus. *Applied physiology, nutrition, and metabolism = Physiologie appliquee, nutrition et metabolisme, 40*(8), 755–761. https://doi.org/10.1139/apnm-2014-0530

Bopp, M. et al. (2008). Lean mass loss is associated with low protein intake during dietary-induced weight loss in postmenopausal women. *Journal of the American Dietetic Association, 108*(7), 1216–1220. https://doi.org/10.1016/j.jada.2008.04.017 https://doi.org/10.1016/j.jada.2008.04.017

Bowen, J. (2019). *The role of protein for health.* CSIRO Proteins for Food and Health Seminar Series March 2019 (Presentation)

Clifton, P. et al. (2009). High protein diets decrease total and abdominal fat and improve CVD risk profile in overweight and obese men and women with elevated triacylglycerol. *Nutrition, metabolism, and cardiovascular diseases, 19*(8), 548–554. https://doi.org/10.1016/j.numecd.2008.10.006

Gordon, M. et al. (2008). Effects of dietary protein on the composition of weight loss in post-menopausal women. *The journal of nutrition, health & aging, 12*(8), 505–509. https://doi.org/10.1007/BF02983202

Pesta, D., & Samuel, V. (2014). A high-protein diet for reducing body fat: mechanisms and possible caveats. *Nutrition & metabolism, 11*(1), 53. https://doi.org/10.1186/1743-7075-11-53

Weigle, D. et al. (2005). A high-protein diet induces sustained reductions in appetite, ad libitum caloric intake, and body weight despite compensatory changes in diurnal plasma leptin and ghrelin concentrations. *The American journal of clinical nutrition, 82*(1), 41–48. https://doi.org/10.1093/ajcn.82.1.41

Westerterp, K. (2004). Diet induced thermogenesis. *Nutrition & metabolism, 1*(1), 5. https://doi.org/10.1186/1743-7075-1-5

Fat

Nutrient Reference Values for Australia and New Zealand. Fats: Total fat and fatty acids https://www.nrv.gov.au/nutrients/fats-total-fat-fatty-acids

Opie, R. et al. (2017). Dietary recommendations for the prevention of depression. *Nutritional neuroscience, 20*(3), 161–171. https://doi.org/10.1179/1476830515Y.0000000043

Saturated fat

Astrup, A. et al. (2020). Saturated fats and health: a reassessment and proposal for food-based recommendations: JACC state-of-the-art review. *Journal of the American College of Cardiology, 76*(7), 844–857. https://doi.org/10.1016/j.jacc.2020.05.077

*Ho, F. et al. (2020). Associations of fat and carbohydrate intake with cardiovascular disease and mortality: prospective cohort study of UK Biobank participants. *BMJ (Clinical research ed.), 368*, m688. https://doi.org/10.1136/bmj.m688

Kris-Etherton, P. et al. (2018). Convincing evidence supports reducing saturated fat to decrease cardiovascular disease risk. *BMJ nutrition, prevention & health, 1*(1), 23–26. https://doi.org/10.1136/bmjnph-2018-000009

*Sacks, F. et al (2017). Dietary fats and cardiovascular disease: a presidential advisory from the American Heart Association. *Circulation;136,3:*e1-e23 https://www.ahajournals.org/doi/epub/10.1161/CIR.0000000000000510

*Tutunchi, H. et al. (2020). The effects of diets enriched in monounsaturated oleic acid on the management and prevention of obesity: a systematic review of human intervention studies. *Advances in nutrition (Bethesda, Md.)*, *11*(4), 864–877 https://doi.org/10.1093/advances/nmaa013

Omega-3 vs. Omega-6 and processed vegetable oils

DiNicolantonio, J., & O'Keefe, J. (2018). Omega-6 vegetable oils as a driver of coronary heart disease: the oxidized linoleic acid hypothesis. *Open heart*, *5*(2), e000898. https://doi.org/10.1136/openhrt-2018-000898

Jenkinson, A. (2020). *Why we eat (too much). The new science of appetite.* Penguin (2020)

Neelakantan, N. et al. (2020). The effect of coconut oil consumption on cardiovascular risk factors: a systematic review and meta-analysis of clinical trials. *Circulation. 2020;141*:803–814 https://www.ahajournals.org/doi/10.1161/CIRCULATIONAHA.119.043052

Trans fats

World Health Organization. (2018). REPLACE trans fat: frequently asked questions. World Health Organization. https://apps.who.int/iris/handle/10665/331304

*Wu, J. et al. (2017). Levels of trans fats in the food supply and population consumption in Australia: an Expert Commentary rapid review brokered by the Sax Institute (www.saxinstitute.org.au) for The National Heart Foundation of Australia, 2017. https://www.heartfoundation.org.au/getmedia/e27233c8-73d5-4c37-9416-ad7592af593c/Expert-Commentary-Levels-of-trans-fats-in-the-food-supply-and-consumption-in-Australia.pdf

Refined fats and overheated or repeated deep-frying

Wu, Y. et al. (2019). The effect of refining process on the physicochemical properties and micronutrients of rapeseed oils. *PLoS ONE 14*(3): e0212879. https://doi.org/10.1371/journal.pone.0212879

Guillaume, C. et al. (2018). Evaluation of chemical and physical changes in different commercial oils during heating. *Acta Scientific Nutritional Health 2*(6): 02-11. https://actascientific.com/ASNH/pdf/ASNH-02-0083.pdf

Perumalla Venkata, R., & Subramanyam, R. (2016). Evaluation of the deleterious health effects of consumption of repeatedly heated vegetable oil. *Toxicology reports*, *3*, 636–643. https://doi.org/10.1016/j.toxrep.2016.08.003

Nuts

Grundy, M. et al. (2016). A review of the impact of processing on nutrient bioaccessibility and digestion of almonds. *International journal of food science & technology, 51*(9), 1937–1946. https://doi.org/10.1111/ijfs.13192

*Taylor, H. et al. (2018). The effects of 'activating' almonds on consumer acceptance and gastrointestinal tolerance. *European journal of nutrition, 57*(8), 2771-2783. https://doi.org/10.1007/s00394-017-1543-7

*Kumari, S. et al. (2020). Does 'activating' nuts affect nutrient bioavailability?. *Food chemistry, 319*, 126529. https://doi.org/10.1016/j.foodchem.2020.126529

Carbs

Carbs at the right time (low after lunch)

Kessler, K. et al. (2017). The effect of diurnal distribution of carbohydrates and fat on glycaemic control in humans: a randomized controlled trial. *Scientific reports, 7*, 44170. https://doi.org/10.1038/srep44170

Sugar, danger zone food and their implication in addictive-like eating behaviours

DiFeliceantonio, A. et al. (2018). Supra-additive effects of combining fat and carbohydrate on food reward. *Cell metabolism, 28*(1), 33–44.e3. https://doi.org/10.1016/j.cmet.2018.05.018

Fazzino, T. et al. (2019). Hyper-palatable foods: development of a quantitative definition and application to the US Food System Database. *Obesity, 27*: 1761-1768. https://doi.org/10.1002/oby.22639

Gearhardt, A., & Hebebrand, J. (2021). The concept of "food addiction" helps inform the understanding of overeating and obesity: Debate consensus. *The American journal of clinical nutrition, 113*(2), 274–276. https://doi.org/10.1093/ajcn/nqaa345

Gordon, E. et al. (2018). What is the evidence for "food addiction?" A systematic review. *Nutrients, 10*(4),477. https://doi.org/10.3390/nu10040477

Hu, T. et al. (2012). Effects of low-carbohydrate diets versus low-fat diets on metabolic risk factors: a meta-analysis of randomized controlled clinical trials. *American journal of epidemiology, 176* Suppl 7(Suppl 7), S44–S54. https://doi.org/10.1093/aje/kws264

Schulte, E. et al. (2015). Which foods may be addictive? The roles of processing, fat content, and glycemic load. *PLoS ONE, 10*(2), e0117959. https://doi.org/10.1371/journal.pone.0117959

Fibre

Aoun, A. et al. (2020). The influence of the gut microbiome on obesity in adults and the role of probiotics, prebiotics, and synbiotics for weight loss. *Preventive nutrition and food science, 25*(2), 113–123. https://doi.org/10.3746/pnf.2020.25.2.113

McRorie, J. W., Jr (2015). Evidence-based approach to fiber supplements and clinically meaningful health benefits, Part 1: What to look for and how to recommend an effective fiber therapy. *Nutrition today, 50*(2), 82–89. https://doi.org/10.1097/NT.0000000000000082

McRorie, J. W., Jr (2015b). Evidence-based approach to fiber supplements and clinically meaningful health benefits, Part 2: What to look for and how to recommend an effective fiber therapy. *Nutrition today, 50*(2), 90-97. https://doi.org/10.1097/NT.0000000000000082

Mills, S. et al. (2019). Precision nutrition and the microbiome, Part I: Current state of the science. *Nutrients, 11*(4), 923. https://doi.org/10.3390/nu11040923

Mills, S. et al. (2019). Precision nutrition and the microbiome, Part II: Potential opportunities and pathways to commercialisation. *Nutrients, 11*(7):1468. https://doi.org/10.3390/nu11071468

Sawicki, C. et al. (2021). Comparison of indices of carbohydrate quality and food sources of dietary fiber on longitudinal changes in waist circumference in the Framingham Offspring Cohort. *Nutrients, 13*(3), 997. https://doi.org/10.3390/nu13030997

Sugar

Casperson, S. et al. (2019). Increasing chocolate's sugar content enhances its psychoactive effects and intake. *Nutrients, 11*(3), 596. https://doi.org/10.3390/nu11030596

Faruque, S. et al. (2019). The dose makes the poison: sugar and obesity in the United States - a review. *Polish journal of food and nutrition sciences, 69*(3), 219–233. https://doi.org/10.31883/pjfns/110735

Stanhope, K. (2016). Sugar consumption, metabolic disease and obesity: The state of the controversy. *Critical reviews in clinical laboratory sciences, 53*(1), 52–67. https://doi.org/10.3109/10408363.2015.1084990

Non-sugar sweeteners

Azad, M. et al. (2017). Nonnutritive sweeteners and cardiometabolic health: a systematic review and meta-analysis of randomized controlled trials and prospective cohort studies. *CMAJ : Canadian Medical Association journal, 189*(28), E929–E939. https://doi.org/10.1503/cmaj.161390

Higgins, K., & Mattes, R. (2019). A randomized controlled trial contrasting the effects of 4 low-calorie sweeteners and sucrose on body weight in adults with overweight or obesity. *The American journal of clinical nutrition, 109*(5), 1288–1301. https://doi.org/10.1093/ajcn/nqy381

Shrapnel, W., & Butcher, B. (2020). Sales of sugar-sweetened beverages in Australia: A trend analysis from 1997 to 2018. *Nutrients, 12*(4), 1016. https://doi.org/10.3390/nu12041016

Tucker, R., & Tan, S. (2017). Do non-nutritive sweeteners influence acute glucose homeostasis in humans? A systematic review. *Physiology & behavior, 182*, 17–26. https://doi.org/10.1016/j.physbeh.2017.09.016

Turner, A. et al. (2020). Intense sweeteners, taste receptors and the gut microbiome: A metabolic health perspective. *International journal of environmental research and public health, 17*(11), 4094. https://www.mdpi.com/1660-4601/17/11/4094

Yang, Q. (2010). Gain weight by 'going diet'? Artificial sweeteners and the neurobiology of sugar cravings. *The Yale journal of biology and medicine, 83*(2):101 – 108. https://www.ncbi.nlm.nih.gov/pmc/articles/PMC2892765/

Fructose

Pollock, N. et al. (2012). Greater fructose consumption is associated with cardiometabolic risk markers and visceral adiposity in adolescents. *The Journal of nutrition, 142*(2), 251–257. https://doi.org/10.3945/jn.111.150219

CHAPTER FIVE. WHAT TO DRINK

Water

Chang, T. et al. (2016). Inadequate hydration, BMI, and obesity among US adults: NHANES 2009-2012. *Annals of family medicine, 14*(4), 320–324. https://doi.org/10.1370/afm.1951

Daniels, M., & Popkin, B. (2010). Impact of water intake on energy intake and weight status: a systematic review. *Nutrition reviews, 68*(9), 505–521. https://doi.org/10.1111/j.1753-4887.2010.00311.x

Dennis, E. et al. (2009). Beverage consumption and adult weight management: a review. *Eating behaviors, 10*(4), 237-246. https://doi.org/10.1016/j.eatbeh.2009.07.006

*Dennis, E. et al. (2010). Water consumption increases weight loss during a hypocaloric diet intervention in middle-aged and older adults. *Obesity (Silver Spring, Md.), 18*(2), 300–307. https://doi.org/10.1038/oby.2009.235

Dubnov-Raz, G. et al. (2011). Influence of water drinking on resting energy expenditure in overweight children. *International journal of obesity (2005), 35*(10), 1295–1300. https://doi.org/10.1038/ijo.2011.130

Keller, U. et al. (2003). Effects of changes in hydration on protein, glucose and lipid metabolism in man: impact on health. *European journal of clinical nutrition, 57 Suppl 2*, S69–S74. https://doi.org/10.1038/sj.ejcn.1601904

Liska, D. et al. (2019). Narrative review of hydration and selected health outcomes in the general population. *Nutrients, 11*(1), 70. https://doi.org/10.3390/nu11010070

*Pan, A. et al. (2013). Changes in water and beverage intake and long-term weight changes: results from three prospective cohort studies. *International journal of obesity (2005), 37*(10), 1378–1385. https://doi.org/10.1038/ijo.2012.225

*Pan, X. et al. (2020). Plain water intake and association with the risk of overweight in the Chinese adult population: China Health and Nutrition Survey 2006-2011. *Journal of epidemiology, 30*(3), 128–135. https://doi.org/10.2188/jea.JE20180223

*Parretti, H. et al. (2015). Efficacy of water preloading before main meals as a strategy for weight loss in primary care patients with obesity: RCT. *Obesity (Silver Spring, Md.), 23*(9), 1785–1791. https://doi.org/10.1002/oby.21167

RACGP (2013). Handbook of Non Drug Intervention (HANDI) Pre-meal water consumption for weight. *Australian Family Physician vol 42* no 6, June 2013 https://www.racgp.org.au/afp/2013/july/pre-meal-water/

*Sedaghat, G. et al. (2021). Effect of pre-meal water intake on the serum levels of Copeptin, glycemic control, lipid profile and anthropometric indices in patients with type 2 diabetes mellitus: a randomized, controlled trial. *Journal of diabetes and metabolic disorders, 20*(1), 171–177. https://doi.org/10.1007/s40200-020-00724-9

Stookey, J. et al. (2014). Qualitative and/or quantitative drinking water recommendations for pediatric obesity treatment. *Journal of obesity & weight loss therapy, 4*(4), 232. https://doi.org/10.4172/2165-7904.1000232

Stookey, J. (2016). Negative, null and beneficial effects of drinking water on energy intake, energy expenditure, fat oxidation and weight change in randomised trials: A qualitative review. *Nutrients, 8*(1), 19. https://doi.org/10.3390/nu8010019

*Stookey, J. et al. (2020). Underhydration is associated with obesity, chronic diseases, and death within 3 to 6 years in the U.S. population aged 51-70 years. *Nutrients, 12*(4), 905. https://doi.org/10.3390/nu12040905

Vij, V., & Joshi, A. (2013). Effect of 'water induced thermogenesis' on body weight, body mass index and body composition of overweight subjects. *Journal of clinical and diagnostic research : JCDR, 7*(9), 1894–1896. https://doi.org/10.7860/JCDR/2013/5862.3344

*Vij, V., & Joshi, A. (2014). Effect of excessive water intake on body weight, body mass index, body fat, and appetite of overweight female participants. *Journal of natural science, biology, and medicine, 5*(2), 340–344. https://pubmed.ncbi.nlm.nih.gov/25097411/

Walton, J. et al. (2019). Cross-sectional association of dietary water intakes and sources, and adiposity: National Adult Nutrition Survey, the Republic of Ireland. *European journal of nutrition, 58*(3), 1193–1201. https://doi.org/10.1007/s00394-018-1635-z

Caffeine

Killer, S. et al. (2014). No evidence of dehydration with moderate daily coffee intake: a counterbalanced cross-over study in a free-living population. *PLoS ONE, 9*(1), e84154. https://doi.org/10.1371/journal.pone.0084154

O'Callaghan, F. et al. (2018). Effects of caffeine on sleep quality and daytime functioning. *Risk management and healthcare policy, 11*, 263–271. https://doi.org/10.2147/RMHP.S156404

Green tea

Prasanth, M. et al. (2019). A review of the role of green tea (camellia sinensis) in antiphotoaging, stress resistance, neuroprotection, and autophagy. *Nutrients, 11*(2), 474. https://doi.org/10.3390/nu11020474

Liu, K. et al. (2013). Effect of green tea on glucose control and insulin sensitivity: a meta-analysis of 17 randomized controlled trials. *The American journal of clinical nutrition, 98*(2), 340–348. https://doi.org/10.3945/ajcn.112.052746

Alkaline water

Fenton, T., & Huang, T. (2016). Systematic review of the association between dietary acid load, alkaline water and cancer. *BMJ open, 6*(6), e010438. https://doi.org/10.1136/bmjopen-2015-010438

Vinegar

*Cheng, L. et al. (2020). A systematic review and meta-analysis: Vinegar consumption on glycaemic control in adults with type 2 diabetes mellitus. *Journal of advanced nursing, 76*(2), 459–474. https://doi.org/10.1111/jan.14255

* Kandylis, P. et al. (2021). Health promoting properties of cereal vinegars. *Foods (Basel, Switzerland), 10*(2), 344. https://doi.org/10.3390/foods10020344

*Kondo, T. et al. (2009). Vinegar intake reduces body weight, body fat mass, and serum triglyceride levels in obese Japanese subjects. *Bioscience, biotechnology, and biochemistry, 73*(8), 1837–1843. https://doi.org/10.1271/bbb.90231

Alcohol

Badrick, E. et al. (2008). The relationship between alcohol consumption and cortisol secretion in an aging cohort. *The Journal of clinical endocrinology and metabolism, 93*(3), 750–757. https://doi.org/10.1210/jc.2007-0737

National Health and Medical Research Council. (2009). *Australian Guidelines to reduce health risks from drinking alcohol.* NHMRC, Australia. https://www.nhmrc.gov.au/about-us/publications/australian-guidelines-reduce-health-risks-drinking-alcohol

CHAPTER SIX. HOW TO EAT

Environmental costs of highly processed food

Fardet, A., & Rock, E. (2020). Ultra-processed foods and food system sustainability: what are the links? *Sustainability, 12*(15):6280. https://doi.org/10.3390/su12156280

National Health and Medical Research Council. (2013). *Australian Dietary Guidelines. Appendix G: Food, nutrition and environmental sustainability.* NHMRC, Australia. https://www.eatforhealth.gov.au/sites/default/files/files/the_guidelines/n55_australian_dietary_guidelines.pdf

Swinburn, B. et al. (2019). The global syndemic of obesity, undernutrition, and climate change: The Lancet Commission report. *Lancet (London, England), 393*(10173), 791–846. https://doi.org/10.1016/S0140-6736(18)32822-8

Vega Mejia, N. et al. (2018). Implications of the Western diet for agricultural production, health and climate change. *Frontiers in sustainable food systems, 2*(88). https://doi.org/10.3389/fsufs.2018.00088

*Willett, W. et al. (2019). Food in the Anthropocene: The EAT-Lancet Commission on healthy diets from sustainable food systems. *Lancet (London, England), 393*(10170), 447–492. https://doi.org/10.1016/S0140-6736(18)31788-4

Mindful eating and chewing

Andrade, A. et al. (2008). Eating slowly led to decreases in energy intake within meals in healthy women. *Journal of the American Dietetic Association, 108*(7), 1186–1191. https://doi.org/10.1016/j.jada.2008.04.026

*Argyrakopoulou, G. et al. (2020). How important is eating rate in the physiological response to food intake, control of body weight, and glycemia?. *Nutrients, 12*(6), 1734. https://doi.org/10.3390/nu12061734

Daubenmier, J. et al (2011). Mindfulness intervention for stress eating to reduce cortisol and abdominal fat among overweight and obese women: an exploratory randomized controlled study. *Journal of obesity, 2011*, 651936. https://doi.org/10.1155/2011/651936

Davidson, T. et al. (2019). The cognitive control of eating and body weight: it's more than what you "think". *Frontiers in psychology, 10*, 62. https://doi.org/10.3389/fpsyg.2019.00062

*Dunn, C. et al. (2018). Mindfulness approaches and weight loss, weight maintenance, and weight regain. *Current obesity reports, 7*(1), 37–49. https://doi.org/10.1007/s13679-018-0299-6

Goh, A. et al. (2021). Increased oral processing and a slower eating rate increase glycaemic, insulin and satiety responses to a mixed meal tolerance test. *European journal of nutrition, 60*(5), 2719–2733. https://doi.org/10.1007/s00394-020-02466-z

Hamada, Y., & Hayashi, N. (2021) Chewing increases postprandial diet-induced thermogenesis. *Scientific reports 11*, 23714. https://doi.org/10.1038/s41598-021-03109-x

Morillo Sarto, H. et al. (2019). Efficacy of a mindful-eating programme to reduce emotional eating in patients suffering from overweight or obesity in primary care settings: a cluster-randomised trial protocol. *BMJ open, 9*(11), e031327. https://pubmed.ncbi.nlm.nih.gov/31753880/

Niemeier, H. et al. (2012). An acceptance-based behavioral intervention for weight loss: a pilot study. *Behavior therapy, 43*(2), 427–435. https://doi.org/10.1016/j.beth.2011.10.005

Slyper, A. (2021). Oral processing, satiation and obesity: overview and hypotheses. *Diabetes, metabolic syndrome and obesity : targets and therapy, 14*, 3399–3415. https://doi.org/10.2147/DMSO.S314379

Vargas-Alvarez, M. et al. (2021). Impact of portion control tools on portion size awareness, choice and intake: systematic review and meta-analysis. *Nutrients, 13*(6), 1978. https://doi.org/10.3390/nu13061978

CHAPTER SEVEN. MICRONUTRIENTS, MICROBIOME AND METABOLISM

Micronutrients

*Armborst, D. et al. (2018). Impact of a specific amino acid composition with micronutrients on well-being in subjects with chronic psychological stress and exhaustion conditions: a pilot study. *Nutrients, 10*(5), 551. https://doi.org/10.3390/nu10050551

*Brisebois, S. et al. (2018). Proton pump inhibitors: review of reported risks and controversies. *Laryngoscope investigative otolaryngology, 3*(6), 457-462. https://doi.org/10.1002/lio2.187

Cuciureanu, M., & Vink, R. (2011). Magnesium and stress. In R. Vink (Eds.) et. al., *Magnesium in the Central Nervous System.* University of Adelaide Press. https://www.ncbi.nlm.nih.gov/books/NBK507250/

DiNicolantonio, J. et al. (2018). Subclinical magnesium deficiency: a principal driver of cardiovascular disease and a public health crisis. *Open heart, 5*(1), e000668. https://doi.org/10.1136/openhrt-2017-000668

Eby, G. et al. (2011). Magnesium and major depression. In R. Vink (Eds.) et. al., *Magnesium in the Central Nervous System.* University of Adelaide Press. https://www.ncbi.nlm.nih.gov/books/NBK507250/

Gröber, U. (2019). Magnesium and Drugs. *International journal of molecular sciences, 20*(9), 2094. https://doi.org/10.3390/ijms20092094

Jahnen-Dechent, W., & Ketteler, M. (2012). Magnesium basics. *Clinical kidney journal, 5(Suppl 1),* i3–i14. https://doi.org/10.1093/ndtplus/sfr163

*Marles, R. (2017). Mineral nutrient composition of vegetables, fruits and grains: The context of reports of apparent historical declines. *Journal of food composition and analysis 56;*93–103. https://doi.org/10.1016/j.jfca.2016.11.012

Williamson, G. (2017). The role of polyphenols in modern nutrition. *Nutrition bulletin, 42*(3), 226–235. https://doi.org/10.1111/nbu.12278

Microbiome

*Aoun, A. et al. (2020). The influence of the gut microbiome on obesity in adults and the role of probiotics, prebiotics, and synbiotics for weight loss. *Preventive nutrition and food science, 25*(2), 113–123. https://pubmed.ncbi.nlm.nih.gov/32676461/

*Cerdó, T. et al. (2019). The role of probiotics and prebiotics in the prevention and treatment of obesity. *Nutrients, 11*(3), 635. https://doi.org/10.3390/nu11030635

Dimidi, E. et al. (2019). Fermented foods: definitions and characteristics, impact on the gut microbiota and effects on gastrointestinal health and disease. *Nutrients, 11*(8), 1806. https://doi.org/10.3390/nu11081806

Faruque, S. et al. (2019). The dose makes the poison: sugar and obesity in the United States - a review. *Polish journal of food and nutrition sciences, 69*(3), 219–233. https://doi.org/10.31883/pjfns/110735

Hills, R. et al. (2019). Gut microbiome: profound implications for diet and disease. *Nutrients, 11*(7), 1613. https://doi.org/10.3390/nu11071613

Holscher, H. (2017). Dietary fiber and prebiotics and the gastrointestinal microbiota. *Gut microbes, 8*(2), 172–184. https://doi.org/10.1080/19490976.2017.1290756

McFarland, L. (2014). Use of probiotics to correct dysbiosis of normal microbiota following disease or disruptive events: a systematic review. *BMJ open, 4*(8), e005047. https://doi.org/10.1136/bmjopen-2014-005047

Mills, S. et al. (2019). Precision nutrition and the microbiome Part II: potential opportunities and pathways to commercialisation. *Nutrients, 11*(7):1468. https://doi.org/10.3390/nu11071468

Rodríguez, M. et al. (2015). Obesity changes the human gut mycobiome. *Scientific reports. 5,* 14600. https://doi.org/10.1038/srep14600

*Singh, R. et al. (2017). Influence of diet on the gut microbiome and implications for human health. *Journal of translational medicine, 15*(1), 73. https://doi.org/10.1186/s12967-017-1175-y

*Stavropoulou, E., & Bezirtzoglou, E. (2020). Probiotics in medicine: a long debate. *Frontiers in immunology, 11,* 2192. https://doi.org/10.3389/fimmu.2020.02192

Stiemsma, L. et al. (2020). Does consumption of fermented foods modify the human gut microbiota?. *The Journal of nutrition, 150*(7), 1680–1692. https://doi.org/10.1093/jn/nxaa077

Turner, A. et al. (2020). Intense sweeteners, taste receptors and the gut microbiome. *International journal of environmental research and public health, 17*(11), 4094. https://doi.org/10.3390/ijerph17114094

Voigt, R. et al. (2014). Circadian disorganization alters intestinal microbiota. *PLoS ONE, 9*(5), e97500. https://doi.org/10.1371/journal.pone.0097500

Metabolism

Calcagno, M. et al. (2019). The thermic effect of food: a review. *Journal of the American College of Nutrition.* http://dx.doi.org/10.1080/07315724.2018.1552544

Connolly, J. et al. (1999). Selections from current literature: effects of dieting and exercise on resting metabolic rate and implications for weight management. *Family practice, 16*(2), 196–201. https://doi.org/10.1093/fampra/16.2.196

Fothergill, E. et al. (2016). Persistent metabolic adaptation 6 years after "The Biggest Loser" competition. *Obesity (Silver Spring, Md.), 24*(8), 1612–1619. https://doi.org/10.1002/oby.21538

*Lichtenbelt, W. et al. (2014). Cold exposure--an approach to increasing energy expenditure in humans. *Trends in endocrinology and metabolism, 25*(4), 165–167. https://doi.org/10.1016/j.tem.2014.01.001

MacKenzie-Shalders, K. et al. (2020). The effect of exercise interventions on resting metabolic rate: A systematic review and meta-analysis. *Journal of sports sciences, 38*(14), 1635–1649. https://doi.org/10.1080/02640414.2020.1754716

Richter, J. et al. (2020). Twice as high diet-induced thermogenesis after breakfast vs dinner on high-calorie as well as low-calorie meals. *The Journal of clinical endocrinology and metabolism, 105*(3). https://doi.org/10.1210/clinem/dgz311

Westerterp, K. (2004). Diet induced thermogenesis. *Nutrition & metabolism, 1*(1), 5. https://doi.org/10.1186/1743-7075-1-5

Whiting, S. et al. (2012). Capsaicinoids and capsinoids. A potential role for weight management? A systematic review of the evidence. *Appetite, 59*(2), 341–348. https://doi.org/10.1016/j.appet.2012.05.015

CHAPTER EIGHT. STRESS, SLEEP AND SHIFT WORK

Stress

*Armborst, D. et al. (2018). Impact of a specific amino acid composition with micronutrients on well-being in subjects with chronic psychological stress and exhaustion conditions: a pilot study. *Nutrients, 10*(5), 551. https://doi.org/10.3390/nu10050551

Blaine, S. et al. (2016). Alcohol effects on stress pathways: impact on craving and relapse risk. *Canadian journal of psychiatry 61*(3), 145–153. https://doi.org/10.1177/0706743716632512

De Ridder, D. et al. (2016). The brain, obesity and addiction: an EEG neuroimaging study. *Scientific reports, 6*, 34122. https://doi.org/10.1038/srep34122

*Duong, M. et al. (2012). High cortisol levels are associated with low quality food choice in type 2 diabetes. *Endocrine, 41*(1), 76–81. https://pubmed.ncbi.nlm.nih.gov/21983796/

Hansen, M. et al. (2017). Shinrin-yoku (forest bathing) and nature therapy: a state-of-the-art review. *International journal of environmental research and public health, 14*(8), 851. https://doi.org/10.3390/ijerph14080851

Lovallo, W. et al. (2006). Cortisol responses to mental stress, exercise, and meals following caffeine intake in men and women. *Pharmacology, biochemistry, and behavior, 83*(3), 441–447. https://doi.org/10.1016/j.pbb.2006.03.005

*van der Valk, E. et al. (2018). Stress and obesity: are there more susceptible individuals?. *Current obesity reports, 7*(2), 193–203. https://link.springer.com/article/10.1007/s13679-018-0306-y

Yau, Y., & Potenza, M. (2013). Stress and eating behaviors. *Minerva endocrinologica, 38*(3), 255–267. https://pubmed.ncbi.nlm.nih.gov/24126546/

Young, L. et al.(2019). A systematic review and meta-analysis of B vitamin supplementation on depressive symptoms, anxiety, and stress: effects on healthy and 'at-risk' individuals. *Nutrients, 11*(9), 2232. https://doi.org/10.3390/nu11092232

Sleep

*Adams, R. et al. (2017). Sleep health of Australian adults in 2016: results of the 2016 Sleep Health Foundation national survey. *Sleep health, 3*(1), 35–42. https://doi.org/10.1016/j.sleh.2016.11.005

Briançon-Marjollet, A. et al. (2015). The impact of sleep disorders on glucose metabolism: endocrine and molecular mechanisms. *Diabetology & metabolic syndrome, 7*, 25. https://doi.org/10.1186/s13098-015-0018-3

Cipolla-Neto, J. et al. (2014). Melatonin, energy metabolism, and obesity: a review. *Journal of pineal research, 56*(4), 371–381. https://doi.org/10.1111/jpi.12137

Cuciureanu, M., & Vink, R. (2011). Magnesium and stress. In R. Vink (Eds.) et. al., *Magnesium in the Central Nervous System*. University of Adelaide Press. https://www.ncbi.nlm.nih.gov/books/NBK507250/

Mohd Azmi, N. et al. (2020). Consequences of circadian disruption in shift workers on chrononutrition and their psychosocial well-being. *International journal of environmental research and public health, 17*(6), 2043. https://doi.org/10.3390/ijerph17062043

Noh, J. (2018). The effect of circadian and sleep disruptions on obesity risk. *Journal of obesity & metabolic syndrome, 27*(2), 78–83. https://doi.org/10.7570/jomes.2018.27.2.78

Stein, M., & Friedmann, P. (2005). Disturbed sleep and its relationship to alcohol use. *Substance abuse, 26*(1), 1–13. https://doi.org/10.1300/j465v26n01_01

Shift work

*Mohd Azmi, N. et al. (2020). Consequences of circadian disruption in shift workers on chrononutrition and their psychosocial well-being. *International journal of environmental research and public health, 17*(6), 2043. https://doi.org/10.3390/ijerph17062043

Phoi, Y., & Keogh, J. (2019). Dietary interventions for night shift workers: a literature review. *Nutrients, 11*(10), 2276. https://doi.org/10.3390/nu11102276

Potter, G., & Wood, T. (2020). The future of shift work: circadian biology meets personalised medicine and behavioural science. *Frontiers in nutrition, 7*, 116. https://doi.org/10.3389/fnut.2020.00116

CHAPTER NINE. THE FEMALE FORM

Pregnancy and the early years

Australian Department of Health (2020). *Clinical Practice Guidelines: Pregnancy Care*. Online at https://www.health.gov.au/resources/pregnancy-care-guidelines/part-d-clinical-assessments/weight-and-body-mass-index

Basak, S. et al. (2021). Maternal supply of both arachidonic and docosahexaenoic acids is required for optimal neurodevelopment. *Nutrients, 13*(6), 2061. https://doi.org/10.3390/nu13062061

Fraser, A. et al. (2010). Association of maternal weight gain in pregnancy with offspring obesity and metabolic and vascular traits in childhood. *Circulation, 121*(23), 2557–2564. https://doi.org/10.1161/CIRCULATIONAHA.109.906081

Godfrey, K. et al. (2017). Influence of maternal obesity on the long-term health of offspring. The Lancet. *Diabetes & endocrinology, 5*(1), 53–64. https://doi.org/10.1016/S2213-8587(16)30107-3

*Gould, J. et al. (2021). The influence of Omega-3 long-chain polyunsaturated fatty acid, docosahexaenoic acid, on child behavioral functioning: a review of randomized controlled trials of DHA supplementation in pregnancy, the neonatal period and infancy. *Nutrients, 13*(2), 415. https://doi.org/10.3390/nu13020415

Grieger, J. et al. (2021). A review of maternal overweight and obesity and its impact on cardiometabolic outcomes during pregnancy and postpartum. *Therapeutic advances in reproductive health, 15*, 2633494120986544. https://doi.org/10.1177/2633494120986544

Jouanne, M. et al. (2021). Nutrient requirements during pregnancy and lactation. *Nutrients, 13*(2), 692. https://doi.org/10.3390/nu13020692

Lauritzen, L. et al. (2016). DHA effects in brain development and function. *Nutrients, 8*(1), 6. https://doi.org/10.3390/nu8010006

*Middleton, P. et al. (2018). Omega-3 fatty acid addition during pregnancy. *The Cochrane database of systematic reviews, 11*(11), CD003402. https://doi.org/10.1002/14651858.CD003402.pub3

*Royal Australian College of General Practitioners (2019). Omega-3 fatty acid addition in pregnancy to reduce the risk of preterm birth. https://www.racgp.org.au/clinical-resources/clinical-guidelines/handi/handi-interventions/nutrition/omega-3-fatty-acid-addition-in-pregnancy-to-reduce

Stubert, J. et al. (2018). The risks associated with obesity in pregnancy. *Deutsches Arzteblatt international, 115*(16), 276–283. https://doi.org/10.3238/arztebl.2018.0276

*Vinding, R. et al. (2018). Effect of fish oil supplementation in pregnancy on bone, lean, and fat mass at six years: randomised clinical trial. *BMJ* 2018; 362: k3312 doi: https://doi.org/10.1136/bmj.k3312

Voerman, E. et al. (2019). Maternal body mass index, gestational weight gain, and the risk of overweight and obesity across childhood: an individual participant data meta-analysis. *PLoS medicine, 16*(2), e1002744. https://doi.org/10.1371/journal.pmed.1002744

Menopause

Beck, V. et al. (2005). Phytoestrogens derived from red clover: an alternative to estrogen replacement therapy?. *The Journal of steroid biochemistry and molecular biology, 94*(5), 499–518. https://doi.org/10.1016/j.jsbmb.2004.12.038

Geraci, A. et al. (2021). Sarcopenia and menopause: the role of estradiol. *Frontiers in endocrinology, 12*, 682012. https://doi.org/10.3389/fendo.2021.682012

*Iyengar, N. et al. (2019). Association of body fat and risk of breast cancer in postmenopausal women with normal body mass index: a secondary analysis of a randomized clinical trial and observational study. *JAMA oncology, 5*(2), 155–163. https://doi.org/10.1001/jamaoncol.2018.5327

Jehan, S. et al. (2017). Sleep, melatonin, and the menopausal transition: what are the links?. *Sleep science (Sao Paulo, Brazil), 10*(1), 11–18. https://doi.org/10.5935/1984-0063.20170003

Kroenke, C. et al. (2012). Effects of a dietary intervention and weight change on vasomotor symptoms in the Women's Health Initiative. *Menopause (New York, N.Y.), 19*(9), 980–988. https://doi.org/10.1097/gme.0b013e31824f606e

Saccomani, S. et al. (2017). Does obesity increase the risk of hot flashes among midlife women?: a population-based study. *Menopause (New York, N.Y.), 24*(9), 1065–1070. https://doi.org/10.1097/GME.0000000000000884

CHAPTER TEN. NAVIGATING THE DAY

Apolzan, J. et al. (2017). Frequency of consuming foods predicts changes in cravings for those foods during weight loss: The POUNDS Lost Study. *Obesity (Silver Spring, Md.), 25*(8), 1343–1348. https://doi.org/10.1002/oby.21895

Gordon, E. et al. (2018). What is the evidence for "food addiction?" A systematic review. *Nutrients, 10*(4), 477. https://doi.org/10.3390/nu10040477

Hitze, B. et al. (2010). How the selfish brain organizes its supply and demand. *Frontiers in neuroenergetics, 2*, 7. https://doi.org/10.3389/fnene.2010.00007

Jacques, A. et al. (2019). The impact of sugar consumption on stress driven, emotional and addictive behaviors. *Neuroscience and biobehavioral reviews, 103*, 178–199. https://doi.org/10.1016/j.neubiorev.2019.05.021

Leidy, H. et al. (2011). The effects of consuming frequent, higher protein meals on appetite and satiety during weight loss in overweight/obese men. *Obesity (Silver Spring, Md.), 19*(4), 818–824. https://doi.org/10.1038/oby.2010.203

Lvovskaya, S., & Smith, D. (2013). A spoonful of bitter helps the sugar response go down. *Neuron, 79*(4), 612–614. https://doi.org/10.1016/j.neuron.2013.07.038

Martin, C. et al. (2011). Change in food cravings, food preferences, and appetite during a low-carbohydrate and low-fat diet. *Obesity (Silver Spring, Md.), 19*(10), 1963–1970. https://doi.org/10.1038/oby.2011.62

Peters, A. et al. (2011). The selfish brain: stress and eating behavior. *Frontiers in neuroscience, 5*, 74. https://doi.org/10.3389/fnins.2011.00074

Rezaie, P. et al. (2021). Effects of bitter substances on GI function, energy intake and glycaemia – do preclinical findings translate to outcomes in humans? *Nutrients 2021, 13(4)*, 1317. https://doi.org/10.3390/nu13041317

Scheer, F. et al. (2013). The internal circadian clock increases hunger and appetite in the evening independent of food intake and other behaviors. *Obesity (Silver Spring, Md.), 21*(3), 421–423. https://doi.org/10.1002/oby.20351

Westerterp-Plantenga, M. et al. (2012). Dietary protein – its role in satiety, energetics, weight loss and health. *The British journal of nutrition, 108 Suppl 2*, S105–S112. https://doi.org/10.1017/S0007114512002589

CHAPTER ELEVEN. WHAT'S COOKING?

Shopping

Harris, J. et al. (2020). Marketing to children in supermarkets: an opportunity for public policy to improve children's diets. *International journal of environmental research and public health, 17*(4), 1284. https://doi.org/10.3390/ijerph17041284

Hecht, A. et al. (2020). Influence of food and beverage companies on retailer marketing strategies and consumer behavior. *International journal of environmental research and public health, 17*(20):7381 https://doi.org/10.3390/ijerph17207381

*Riesenberg, D. et al. (2019). Price promotions by food category and product healthiness in an Australian supermarket chain. *American journal of public health, 109*(10), 1434–1439. https://doi.org/10.2105/AJPH.2019.305229

CHAPTER TWELVE. FOOD ADVERTISING – DON'T BUY IT

Australian Government Department of Health. (2017). *Policy Context Relating to Sugars in Australia and New Zealand*. Australian Government. https://www1.health.gov.au/internet/fr/publishing.nsf/Content/C6995F10A56B5D56CA2581EE00177CA8/$File/Policy%20Context%202017.pdf

*DiFeliceantonio, A. et al. (2018). Supra-additive effects of combining fat and carbohydrate on food reward. *Cell metabolism, 28*(1), 33–44.e3. https://doi.org/10.1016/j.cmet.2018.05.018

Food Regulation Standing Committee. (2019). *Policy Paper: Labelling of sugars on packaged food and drinks*. Food Standards Australia New Zealand (FSANZ). https://foodregulation.gov.au/internet/fr/publishing.nsf/Content/sugar-labelling

Gaesser, G., & Angadi, S. (2012). Gluten-free diet: imprudent dietary advice for the general population?. *Journal of the Academy of Nutrition and Dietetics, 112*(9), 1330–1333. https://doi.org/10.1016/j.jand.2012.06.009

Gordon, E. et al. (2018). What is the evidence for "food addiction?" A systematic review. *Nutrients, 10*(4), 477. https://doi.org/10.3390/nu10040477

Gupta, R. et al. (2020) Endocrine disruption and obesity: a current review on environmental obesogens. *Current research in green and sustainable chemistry, 3*, 100009, ISSN 2666-0865. https://doi.org/10.1016/j.crgsc.2020.06.002

https://www.betreatwise.info/about-be-treatwise/#

Mills, S. et al. (2019). Precision nutrition and the microbiome, Part I: current state of the science. *Nutrients, 11*(4), 923. https://doi.org/10.3390/nu11040923

INDEX

www.ingramcontent.com/pod-product-compliance
Lightning Source LLC
Chambersburg PA
CBHW052009030426
42334CB00029BA/3146